THE
HYPNOBIRTHING
BOOK

An Inspirational Guide for a Calm,
Confident, Natural Birth

Katharine Graves

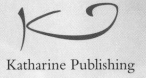

Katharine Publishing

First published in Great Britain in 2012 by:
Katharine Publishing, 50 Fosbury, Marlborough, Wiltshire, SN8 3NJ

The author has made every reasonable effort to contact all copyright holders. Any errors that may have occurred are inadvertent and anyone who for any reason has not been contacted is invited to write to the publisher so that a full acknowledgement may be made in subsequent editions of this work.

British Library Cataloguing in Publication Data
A catalogue record for this book is available from the British Library

ISBN 978-0-9571445-0-7

Editor: Jennifer McIntyre
Art editor and page make-up: Louise Turpin
Cover design: Alex Graham
Illustrations: Fiona McIntyre
Photography: Shutterstock

Printed and bound in the UK by:
ImprintDigital.net, Upton Pyne, Devon, EX5 5HY

This book is designed to provide helpful information on pregnancy and birth. It does not constitute medical advice or an alternative to appropriate medical care, nor is it in any way a guarantee or promise of expected, imagined or actual outcome of labour or birth. It is not a substitute for the advice or the presence during birth or any part of pregnancy or labour of a qualified medical practitioner, midwife or obstetrician. Neither the author nor the publisher accept responsibility for any liability or damage caused by or as a result of practising the techniques in this book.

To Archie McIntyre,
the unsung hero of hypnobirthing

Contents

'According to physiological law, all natural functions of the body are achieved without peril or pain. Birth is a natural, normal physiological function for normal, healthy women and their healthy babies. It can, therefore, be inferred that healthy women, carrying healthy babies, can safely birth without peril or pain.'

Dr Jonathan Dye, *Easier Childbirth*, 1891

Foreword

This excellent hypnobirthing book will reach softly into the hearts and minds of parents approaching birth and fill them with inspirational visions of possibilities and aspirations for beautiful, peaceful, calm births for their babies and for themselves. Katharine's personal qualities – unfailing positivity, humour, the deepest respect for birth and for women, their partners and their babies, and a deep faith in the natural birth process – shine out of the pages of this splendid book.

As a midwife, I provide care to women throughout pregnancy, birth and beyond. Part of the midwife's role is to provide sound evidence-based information for couples about the various available options around birth and the many interventions in the physiological process which have become so routine that they are rarely questioned and, indeed, are widely believed to be true, despite, in some cases, an unsatisfactory or absent evidence base. The midwife then helps the couple to explore the risks and benefits of each intervention and the risks and benefits of declining these interventions, so that they can make an informed plan of their preferences.

Birth, of course, has its own agenda and does not always play out the way we might wish. Hypnobirthing is so important here too, as a calm mother can help her baby even during a complex or challenging birth. As a midwife, I also have a responsibility to inform the woman and her partner about their legal and moral rights in relation to accepting or declining aspects of health care offered to them. Couples empowered by attending Katharine's hypnobirthing courses, and by reading this book, will be in a much stronger position to face this daunting task of making informed plans for pregnancy, birth and new parenting that are right for their family.

In this inspiring book, Katharine's philosophy challenges the widespread and insidious tocophobia (pathological fear of birth) which makes pregnancy and birth so challenging today. It will be an excellent additional resource in the long journey our society needs to take back towards embracing normal birth sensations. Hypnobirthing can, and frequently does, provide a way for a mother and her baby to have a calm, drug-free, gentle and more comfortable birth. Using hypnobirthing techniques, mothers are more in tune with their powerful inner strength and can experience the transformational nature of birth, emerging full of wonder at their new-found exhilaration and sense of their own power. Their babies are born smoothly and simply, requiring fewer of the interventions and medications that can make birth so hazardous for some. Their partners are in tune with the vital work of birth, ready to nurture and protect the mother as she births her child and to receive the baby with joy and love, drawing the new family into embracing and protective arms.

Peace on Earth begins with Birth.

Liz Nightingale
Midwife and hypnobirthing teacher
www.purplewalnutmidwife.co.uk

Introduction

This is the story of how many people arrive at a hypnobirthing class. Before a woman becomes pregnant, she may have at the back of her mind, if she has thought about it at all, that she could always have a Caesarean section as a soft option. Then she becomes pregnant, does some research and realises that a Caesarean is certainly not a soft option; it is major abdominal surgery. Her hormones start to do somersaults, and she begins to realise that a natural birth is better for her and for her baby. Then the mother starts to hear some of the horror stories about birth which people seem to delight in telling pregnant women, and she begins to think that there's only one option and it's going to be painful.

At this point she hears the magic word 'hypnobirthing'. She searches the Internet to find out more, and decides it's a good idea and that she would like to do it. Pregnant women seem to spend their whole life on the Internet – I sometimes wonder how anyone ever managed to have a baby before it existed. She tells her partner that she's thinking of doing hypnobirthing, at which point he raises his eyes to heaven and wonders, 'What is she on to now? She'll only burst into tears again if I object, and we've had so many other expenses, so why do we have to pay for this as well?' And then, even worse, he discovers he is supposed to come to the classes too.

That's the scenario when a great many couples enter the room for the hypnobirthing class.

They come sceptical, and why shouldn't they, because the name implies something that is rather odd and hippyish. With a bit of luck you go into a strange, spaced-out state where hopefully something happens and you don't notice the pain. Nothing could be further from the truth, and hypnobirthing is based on sound and irrefutable logic. People arrive at the class sceptical, and leave enthusiastic and positive.

Probably the most sceptical person I ever taught was my daughter-in-law. She only came to the class because I was her mother-in-law and she couldn't get out of it. On the day her baby was born, she woke up at 6.30am with twinges in her back, but went back to sleep until about 11am. At 1pm they rang the hospital as her contractions were very erratic but coming closer together. The hospital told her to wait until the contractions were regular, five minutes apart and one minute long, and to go and have a nice warm bath and relax, which is hospital speak (in the nicest possible way) to say that she was ringing far too early, as most first-time mothers do, and to go away. She got in the bath at about 2pm and, although the contractions were never a steady five minutes apart, by about 4.15pm she felt the need to push. The two hours or so in between had felt a lot shorter. By 4.30pm she and my son were in a taxi and on their way to hospital. Goodness knows what the driver must have thought seeing a heavily pregnant woman get into his taxi and sit on a towel – as her waters had not yet broken.

They couldn't quite get to the hospital because of roadworks, so they walked through the roadworks and every time my daughter-in-law had a contraction, my son put down her bag and she leant on him and did her breathing exercises, then he picked up her bag again and they went on their way. She remarked that even in the middle of a contraction it was still funny to be standing in the middle of a street just a block from the hospital, trying not to push and give birth then and there. When they reached the hospital she was already fully dilated, there was no time to fill the birthing pool, and the baby was born half an hour later. She says, 'It was an extremely calm experience. My husband was cracking jokes and I was laughing just minutes before the baby was born. There was no pain during and no pain afterwards. The baby didn't cry when he was born, and not very much afterwards either.'

Just to be sure, I asked her later if there was any pain and she said, 'No. No pain.'

My daughter, on the other hand, planned to have her baby at home, but at 43 weeks the baby still hadn't arrived so she finally agreed to an induction. This is no light decision as an induction can make a significant difference to labour. But my daughter went through the whole induced labour using hypnobirthing techniques and with no drugs, which is a massive accolade to her, and to hypnobirthing. At the end, the baby was in distress (as can often happen with an induced labour) so she had a Caesarean section. But hypnobirthing made a difference even in these circumstances. She had no drugs until the spinal block for the Caesarean, and her calm state of mind, rather than feeling stressed, meant that she would have been producing different hormones, which would have made a difference to her and to her baby. (We'll look more at hormones in Chapter 2.)

These are two very different scenarios. We would all like the first, pain-free birth. It can happen, and frequently does with hypnobirthing. The second might not be considered the perfect birth, but hypnobirthing still made a difference. Hypnobirthing cannot promise the perfect pain-free birth, but in my experience, it always makes a difference, and a very big difference too.

CHAPTER 1

Hypnobirthing Explained

'... *Birth is a secret of Nature.*'

Marcus Aurelius,
Meditations, 170–180 AD

Hypnobirthing Explained

Most women come to a hypnobirthing class with their partners; some come on their own. You can do it either way. Fathers often come to the class unwillingly, but by the end are the most enthusiastic advocates of the method and are so glad they came.

Hypnobirthing enables a woman to work with her body, which is naturally designed to give birth. It releases the fear and negativity that she has been programmed with from an early age (everyone knows that birth is painful, don't they?), and replaces it with calm confidence, so she can enjoy this amazing experience of pregnancy and birth.

Hypnotherapy

Some people have used hypnotherapy very effectively to help them stop smoking or cope with a fear of flying, but for many people it is a word that conjures up rather strange images of stage hypnotists making people cluck like a chicken or bark like a dog, or eat an onion thinking it's an apple. In fact, hypnotherapy is merely the use of words: words used in a more focused and positive way to help people let go of some of the negative ideas they have acquired in life. When you stop to think for a moment, our world view as an adult is simply the sum total of all the phrases we have heard and all the experiences we have had throughout our life; most of them are positive, but a few are negative. It's the human condition.

People's response to hypnotherapy is interesting too. I remember I was once working with a lady on weight loss and at the end of the session she said, 'It can't possibly have worked, because I heard every word you said, and I spent the whole time worrying that I hadn't turned off my mobile phone and that it might ring.' Her perception was that in hypnotherapy you have to go into some curious, spaced-out state, and then words waft over you and something happens. The funny thing is that she came back the next week and said, 'It was really strange. I just didn't want to pick at food during the week.' Plainly her mind had been so busy thinking about her mobile phone that the suggestions I had given had slipped in under the radar, and had worked well.

On the other hand, someone else can be so relaxed that they are practically out for the count. They look as if they are asleep, but they are not; they are in hypnosis. But at the end of the session they will probably say, 'It can't possibly have worked because I didn't hear a word you said.' Their assumption is that, in order for anything to happen, the conscious mind has to think about it and process it. But hypnotherapy will work equally well for that person too. And you know they have heard because, at the end of the session, when you suggest they open their eyes and 'come back into the room', they do. So even though they appear to be asleep, something is still listening. It is very interesting.

The power of language

Kipling said that words are the most powerful drug known to man, which is an accurate statement of the power of words.

A word in the right or the wrong place can make or ruin a friendship for life. When I went on holiday last year I remarked to a friend that I was going skiing, and he said. 'Oh, do you still ski?' Now, 'Do you ski?' is an entirely neutral question. 'Do you *still* ski?' means that you look so old and decrepit that I didn't think you could possibly stagger onto a couple of planks and slide down a mountain. I was very polite and I didn't laugh, because if my friend had realised what he had said, he would have been mortified. But his question revealed exactly what he was thinking, and one little word made all the difference.

Similarly, every mother who has been at home looking after a baby or a child will have been asked, 'Do you work, or are you just a housewife?' Now the first question, 'Do you work?' is insulting enough, and the only answer must be, 'I work 24/7. What are your hours?' But the second phrase is devastating. The little word '*just*' turns you from a normal human being of average height and reasonable intelligence into something about 2cm high, without a brain, that someone could trip over without noticing. To maintain your self-respect in the face of such comments can take a considerable mental effort.

Words are very important, and I would like you to do a simple little exercise now. Relax comfortably, and then notice what happens in your body and in your mind when you ask yourself, 'Am I in pain?' Did the thought of pain enter your head when it hadn't been there before? Did you do a quick check to see if there was any discomfort in your body? Did you perhaps notice the slightest tightening of your forehead or your jaw?

Now settle yourself comfortably again and ask yourself, 'Am I quite comfortable?' Maybe the experience was different this time. Perhaps you felt your shoulders drop a little as the tension eased away?

So, fathers, if a midwife comes into the room when your wife or partner is having her baby and asks if she is in pain, please stop her. Tell her that words are important to you, that they have an effect, and ask her not to use that word again. It is part of your role in making sure the mother feels she is in a calm, safe space as she gives birth, and I'll explain why later on. It is a perfectly good word in normal conversation but in labour it is actively harmful. It can make the mother think about having pain when she was not even considering it before, and cause tension and set her on a path of negative responses. One of the most important things that hypnobirthing fathers do is to make sure their partner feels calm and safe, and when I say that I don't just mean with low lights and soft music but, more importantly, feeling calm mentally and emotionally.

A mother sent me this email:

My husband and I participated in your hypnobirthing course and we both found it incredibly useful and inspiring. Since then we have been practising lots.

I am now 39 and a half weeks pregnant and attended a midwife appointment this morning. She told me that my baby was in the 'wrong position', as the baby's back is against my back and that I would therefore have a 'long and painful labour'. She said that I'm still allowed to go ahead with my homebirth, but that it is now likely that I will have to be transferred to hospital for an assisted delivery.

As you can imagine this has got me into a right panic! I am now really worried about the birth (I had previously been looking forward to it) and frightened that I won't be able to cope. I've looked up exercises that I can do to help the baby move into a better position, but I would be incredibly grateful if you could suggest anything else to help with this situation.

Tell a mother that her baby is in the 'wrong position' and the word *wrong – wrong – wrong* is resonating in her subconscious mind – 'There's something wrong with my baby.' Add to this that labour will be 'long and painful'. Then the words 'I'm still *allowed*' tell her that she is not sufficiently intelligent to take advice and make her own decisions but has to do what she's told like a small child. Next she is told that she will probably have to 'be transferred' – not that 'she will transfer', i.e. something she does, but that 'she will be transferred', i.e. it will be done to her. Then she is frightened by the prospect of a forceps or ventouse (vacuum extraction) delivery when she had been planning a natural birth. What more could you say in two sentences to terrify a mother about to give birth?

Anyway, we did some work and restored her calm and confidence. Ten days later I received another email with her birth report:

> I just wanted to let you know that we had our baby on Wednesday morning. A little girl.
>
> Possibly due to the baby lying back to back, I felt the discomfort exclusively in my back, which led to the midwife on the phone initially telling me that I was not in labour. So, to cut a long story short, by the time a midwife came out to me three hours later I was already 7cm dilated … and I ended up having my baby in the birthing pool approximately seven hours after we made that first telephone call.
>
> My waters didn't break at all, which I think must have helped the baby turn right at the last minute, just before she came out. So I think you were right when you said that 'baby knows best'.
>
> Thank you again, Katharine, for all of your love and kindness and support. It was absolutely invaluable during the run-up to the birth.

My comments on this second email are that a back-to-back labour is more likely to be experienced in the back, and the mother talks about discomfort but not pain. I am surprised that the midwife on the phone didn't realise that, with a back-to-back baby, the mother was describing the signs of early labour; but because she didn't realise this, the mother was able to labour undisturbed so labour progressed well and 7cm in three hours is excellent progress for a first baby, regardless of which way it is facing. A labour of seven hours is also good for a first baby. Also, most back-to-back babies turn in labour (as we will see in Chapter 4), and it would have been consoling for the mother if the first midwife had told her this.

This story is an absolutely classic example of the harm careless words can do, and the difference words can make.

Because words are so powerful, hypnobirthing uses them in a slightly different way. The word 'contraction' is made up of hard sounds: a 'c', 't' and 'n'. It is medical jargon, with connotations of pain. So there are other words that can be used instead: wave, rush or surge. My personal preference is 'surge'. It is made up of soft sounds that have a different effect. It conjures up images of the waves of the sea. Everything in nature works in that wavelike movement: the sea, light, sound, the rhythms of the seasons of the year and the hours of the day all move in waves, and certainly the muscles of the uterus in labour do. They start to work, build up to a peak, and slacken off again. So not only does the word 'surge' have a different effect, but it is perhaps a more accurate description of what is going on.

I know that you may feel rather silly and affected when you start to use the word 'surge' instead of 'contraction', but please do it. After a couple of weeks it will feel quite normal. You will see that all these small changes put together make a very big difference.

Hypnobirthing and the mind

Doing hypnobirthing is a little like learning to play a musical instrument. I could tell you how to play the piano in ten minutes, but it wouldn't mean you could do it. If you went to lessons, you would progress. But if you practised between the lessons, you would progress much faster. For some people, buying this book and listening to a relaxation CD is sufficient, but for many people it is not, and they need to do the whole course with a teacher. But nobody can say, until you have your baby, which category you are in.

Hypnobirthing is made up of a lot of simple little things, because you can't be doing with complicated things when you're giving birth. But put together they make a very big difference. The more you practise the things I suggest, the better the outcome.

As you read through this book, you will probably see a great deal of sense in what I say much of the time. But you may also come up against things that you think are not for you. I'm not saying that I'm right and you're wrong. I'm simply suggesting that everything is important and, if you feel you want to reject something, it may be that it makes you feel uncomfortable because it conflicts with an assumption you have made. If this does happen, I would ask you to take a second look. Do some research. Think about it quietly. Look at the matter again with an open mind. Reconsider it in the light of the new information you have found. And then, if you decide to change your mind, that's fine. If you decide your original judgement was right, that's fine too. But you will be coming to that decision from a place of knowledge and not from an assumption based on nothing more than social folklore about having a baby.

When talking about how the mind works, the analogy has been used that the mind is like an iceberg. The conscious mind, the brain, is like the part you can see above the surface of the water. It is large and powerful and should be treated with great respect, and we are hugely privileged to have this amazing tool. But underneath the water is the far larger part of the iceberg, and this part is like the unconscious mind. It is difficult to answer questions about the unconscious mind because those questions come from the conscious mind – the thinking part of the mind, the part above the surface. The conscious mind is different from the unconscious mind, and can never really comprehend it. The unconscious mind is far larger, far more powerful, and should be treated with even greater respect.

Einstein is reported to have said: 'The intuitive mind is a sacred gift and the rational mind is a faithful servant. We have created a society that honours the servant and has forgotten the gift.' We are so busy thinking and working things out in our society, that we sometimes forget we have this more intuitive part of the mind. We see it in animals: anyone who has a pet dog will know that it will probably be sitting on the doormat a few minutes before its owner comes home. The animal somehow knows, and we wonder at it.

But we have these instincts too. We have all had the experience of reaching out a hand to pick up the phone to call someone, maybe someone on the other side of the world whom we haven't spoken to for a couple of years, and just as we reach out, the phone rings and it's that person calling us. It feels so strange when this happens, because we don't understand it, but we've all had that experience and it's an example of the intuitive mind.

Negative thoughts

In the normal course of life, the words we hear go into our conscious mind, are then processed by the unconscious mind, and have an effect right down to a cellular level of our bodies. So while you are pregnant it is very important that the input into your mind is positive. When pregnant women have been under stress – and I mean extreme stress, not just the normal ups and downs of daily life – their babies have not developed very well. We will look at this in more depth a little later on but, between now and when your baby is born, avoid negative input, either thoughts, words or images. For instance, for the rest of your pregnancy, you are in charge of your television's remote control. There is plenty to watch that is positive, funny, educational and light hearted, and you can always look at a DVD if there is nothing suitable on television. Your husband or partner can put off watching horror movies until after your baby is born.

As soon as you became pregnant, you probably found yourself beset by people telling you horror stories about birth. This is actively harmful to you and to your baby, and no-one has the right to harm you in this way. The trouble is that we have been brought up to be polite and listen to what people say before we reply, but in this case please stop them. One mother I taught used to say, 'I'm sorry, I can't be part of this conversation until after my baby is born, so could we have it then?'

Focus on where you want to be. You get what you focus on. If you drive down the road and try to avoid the potholes, what happens? You drive straight into them. If you want to avoid the potholes, you need to focus on the flat parts of the road. It's exactly the same with everything else in life. I'm not suggesting you should be totally unrealistic. Inform yourself well before you decide anything, then, having made the decision, put the negatives out of your mind and focus on where you want to be. That way you are far more likely to get there.

The mind doesn't take in the negative form. What is the image that pops into your head if I say to you, 'Don't think of a pink elephant?' You can't get the thing out of your mind. When we start to notice, it is amazing how often we talk and think in terms of the negative. 'I'm not very good at this.' 'Don't do that.' If we want our other half to bring something home from the shops, how often do we say, 'Don't forget the milk?' 'Don't . . . forget the milk.' It's just like the pink elephant. Then they come home without the milk and we say, 'I asked you to buy some milk,' but you didn't, you actually told them to forget the milk, and they did exactly what you asked. If you really want them to bring home some milk, you will be far more likely to get it if you say, 'Remember the milk.' Start to notice how often you use the negative, and re-programme yourself to use the positive. It makes a difference, and your life will improve immeasurably.

As I have said, all thoughts are taken in by the brain, processed by the unconscious, and affect us right down to a cellular level. But the thoughts you take in last thing at night have eight hours to go on being processed. So it is particularly important that you go to sleep with a calm mind. How many people watch the news and then go to bed? The news is nothing but death and violence and negativity, and if you fill your mind with such negativity just before you go to bed, your sleep will be disturbed, and you will wake feeling less refreshed in the morning. That is why on my hypnobirthing course you are given a CD to listen to last thing at night with positive statements and visualisations about birth. I'll explain this later on too.

How other mammals give birth

When it comes to birth, we could learn a great deal from our fellow mammals. The brain has little to do with the actual process of giving birth. We can't decide when our babies will be born, and we can't decide how our labour will be, though we can do a lot in preparation to affect it. If you have a cat, and you lovingly prepare a nice cosy box with a blanket in it in a warm corner of the kitchen for her to have her kittens, what happens? One day you notice that you haven't seen your cat for a while, so you mount a search and find her under the bed, or outside in the shed, with eight little kittens. She went to a small, safe place on her own where *she* felt comfortable. Not where you thought she ought to be.

If a farmer has his ewes lambing in a barn, he knows that the one who is about to give birth is the one that retires to the furthest corner and becomes very still. It's the nearest she can get in that environment to going to her small, safe place. If he goes into the house to make a cup of tea, there is a birth explosion in his absence, because the ewes feel safer not being observed.

Now please don't think I'm advocating giving birth without medical support; I am certainly not. But I am saying that if we respect our natural instincts, the birth is more likely to go smoothly and naturally. The more experienced your midwife, the less she will do or say.

In the wild, an animal will take herself away on her own to a place where she feels safe to give birth. If she's not sure, the whole process will stop, or even reverse, until she is sure it is a safe place to have her baby.

We know that animals follow their instincts, but we sometimes forget how powerful our instincts are too. We are so busy using our brains that we forget that, in certain circumstances, they have their limitations. We know that we feel safe in some places and not in others. You can go into a house and it feels entirely like home; you go into another house and you know you could never live there because it just doesn't feel right. Your body relaxes when you are at home in your own safe space, somewhere that you feel comfortable and happy.

If you speak to a midwife who has helped mothers give birth at home, she will say it is amazing the number of times she has been with a woman who has given birth in the loo or in the bathroom. It is simply because the mother has gone to her small, safe place where she is generally alone and can shut out the world, so it is a natural place for her to want to be when she is having her baby. It may be a room upstairs, and so other people are outside and down in the road, and the hurly-burly of the world is shut out. The reason that labour so often slows down when a mother goes to hospital is simply that it is a strange place and she is being observed by strangers.

I often wonder how many mothers who arrive at hospital only to be told that they are only 1cm dilated, they are much too early and should go back home, were actually 4 or 5cm dilated when they left home, and it is just the unnatural experience of travelling across town and going to a strange place that has cause the body to tense up so the whole process has reverted. I have a very good midwife friend who tells me of an occasion when she was caring for a mother in hospital who was doing well and was 6cm dilated when she was examined. Shortly after the examination, the senior midwife bustled into the room to check what was going on, examined the mother again, and found she was 3cm dilated. It was the arrival of a stranger; a slight rush (which is stress) that caused the process to reverse. Nobody had been unpleasant, nobody had been unkind, but the body had just said, 'I'm not quite sure about this,' and the whole process had reverted.

CHAPTER 2

The Uterus, and the Fear and Confident Responses

'If one advances confidently in the
direction of his dreams, and endeavours
to live the life which he has imagined,
he will meet with a success unexpected
in the common hours.'

Henry David Thoreau,
Walden; or, Life in the Woods, 1854

The Uterus, and the Fear and Confident Responses

A mother who had recently used hypnobirthing came into a class to tell the couples about her experience. Her baby was born in three hours with no drugs, pain or tearing. Asked, 'Was it painful?', she replied, 'I can honestly say it wasn't *painful*, but I was amazed at how *powerful* it was.' Painful and powerful are different. We know what it feels like to use our muscles powerfully, and it can still be comfortable.

The uterus

L et's look now at a very important part of hypnobirthing: the muscles of the uterus and how they work.

The uterus is effectively a powerful bag of muscles which contains, protects and nourishes your baby. The external muscles of the upper part of the uterus are vertical fibres which work to draw up in a spiral motion in the first stage of labour. The fibres of the middle layer of the uterus are interwoven with blood vessels. The muscles of the inner layer form horizontal hoops around the cervix which, during pregnancy, keep your baby in. In order for your baby to be born, they have to release and open.

During pregnancy the body of the uterus must remain relaxed and stretch in order to accommodate the growing baby, while the cervix must remain firm in order to keep the baby in. In labour, these two functions are reversed. The muscles of the body of the uterus start to work and draw up, and the muscles of the cervix relax and start to open. The two types of muscle work in harmony. Each has a different function.

The two sets of muscles will work in harmony when the labouring mum is calm and relaxed as nature intended. In the first stage of labour, during surges the vertical muscles draw up. The circular muscles relax and draw back and allow this to happen. The cervix thins and opens. You can see the

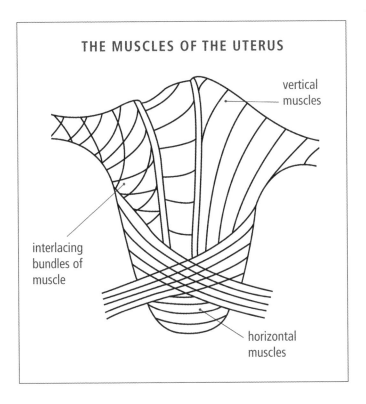

THE MUSCLES OF THE UTERUS

vertical muscles

interlacing bundles of muscle

horizontal muscles

abdomen rising during a surge. I call it the 'up' stage of labour because that is what the muscles are doing.

When I was first told this I thought it was rather odd. How is it that two areas of muscle within the same organ, the uterus, respond in completely different ways to the same message which comes from the hormones and the nervous system? After a while, when I thought it through, I realised that actually it is perfectly logical because all the muscles in the body work in pairs. If you want to do something as simple as bending your arm, the biceps muscle contracts and the triceps muscle releases. The triceps is almost redundant until you want to straighten your arm again, in which case the triceps works and the biceps releases.

All the muscles in the body work in pairs, and so do the muscles of the uterus, which is just as well, because then you have a mechanism for getting back to normal afterwards – the muscles of the cervix contract and the muscles further up release.

The thing is that all the muscles in the body are comfortable doing the job they are designed to do, but the only muscles that are generally considered to be painful are the muscles of the uterus, which seems a most appallingly bad design fault when you consider that these are the muscles which ensure the continuation of the human race. Bear in mind also the miracle that is the human body. When you stop to think for a moment, it is miraculous how the body heals something as simple as a tiny cut. And yet these very important muscles of the uterus are generally considered to be uncomfortable, if not painful, when performing the function they are designed to do. Doesn't this seem rather illogical?

If you have pain in your muscles it is generally because you have taken some unusual and strenuous exercise. If you suddenly went for a 20-mile hike, the muscles in your legs would be painful the next day. If you painted all the ceilings in your home, your arm muscles would be stiff and sore the next day. But nobody ever had labour pains the next day, so this can't be the answer. Now imagine that you had painted all the ceilings in your home, and the next morning when you went to lift something down from a shelf, the movement of your arm would be slow and inefficient and painful simply because, as the biceps muscle went to work, the triceps would be stiff and therefore would not be releasing — so that as you tried to move your arm there would be a battle going on between the two muscles.

It is exactly the same with the muscles of the uterus: as the upper muscles of the uterus work to draw up, if the muscles around the cervix remain tense and do not release, there is a battle between the two sets of muscles. This means that each surge is more uncomfortable, less efficient and longer, there are more of them, and labour is longer. Not only that but, because the muscles are working against each other, they tend to restrict the mother's blood supply. Blood carries oxygen, the primary fuel for each cell in the body, as well as nutrients. For muscle cells to work well they need a good supply of oxygen; so if the oxygen supply to the muscles is restricted, they will work less efficiently.

In addition, the oxygen carried in the mother's blood is the oxygen which goes through the placenta to the baby, so the baby's oxygen supply can be compromised. Therefore the baby is likely to find labour more taxing, so everything is progressing less than optimally.

On the other hand, as the upper muscles of the uterus work to draw up, if the muscles around the cervix gently release with each surge, then each surge is more comfortable, more efficient, shorter, there are fewer of them and labour is shorter.

It's very, very simple, and very, very logical.

The emergency response – the sympathetic nervous system

But then we need to ask the question, 'What tips the mother from the relaxed response to the tense response?' And the answer is . . . fear. The fear response is the way we are designed to deal with emergencies. We call it the sympathetic nervous system. It is a brilliant system that evolved many millennia ago to act as a lifesaver in emergencies, and it works well. But the emergencies we met then were different from the emergencies we meet now. Thousands of years ago you might have been wandering over the brow of a hill and seen a sabre-toothed tiger in the valley in front of you. So what would you do? You freeze – and hope you haven't been seen! If you have been seen you run, and if you can't run fast enough you are obliged to turn and fight. We tend to call it the fight-or-flight response, but actually it's not – it's the freeze-flight-fight response in that order. We all still have it, and it is how we deal with emergencies. The freeze-flight-fight response works in all of us.

The part of this response that is relevant to a woman in labour is the freeze response, because she is not going to be running or fighting. It is the rabbit in the headlights response. It is what happens when you are in a meeting and someone puts you on the spot by asking a difficult question, and you simply can't think of the answer, even though you are aware that you know it perfectly well. And the moment you get home the answer pops into your head, and you say to yourself, 'Why couldn't I have thought of that earlier?' If you play a musical instrument, it's quite likely that your fingers will begin to stumble if someone comes into the room – you're being observed so you tense up. That's the freeze response. The minute you're put under stress, both the mind and the body freeze.

If a mother feels afraid, or even slightly worried or nervous (it doesn't have to be abject terror; it can be quite a minor stress), her body freezes and labour slows down or stops. How often is the cascade of medical interventions started by a stalled labour or a labour that fails to start at all? And what is often the reason for this? Stress, or worry. The human race has survived for millennia because it is a mother's instinct to protect her child, and part of this instinct programmes her to be in a small dark place, hidden away, where she feels absolutely safe before her body is prepared to release her baby and give birth. If she feels under stress, the body simply doesn't work.

No animal will leave a trace of itself in a strange place if it can possibly help it; there might be a predator around. We know this perfectly well. If you go away for a weekend, staying in a beautiful place, very often you will become just a little bit constipated, and the body will not release until you are home again. Or you can be coming home from work, by car or walking down the road, thinking of this and that, and the minute you enter your own front door you need a pee. It's simply due to a natural mental and physical relaxation from being in your home, your own safe place. A baby is a very large and important part of ourselves. How much more careful will a mother's body be in choosing where she expels her baby compared with where she is prepared to expel her normal bodily excretions? It is our instinct to protect our young from predators.

So when a mother feels fearful, what happens? The hormones she produces are affected. The hormones of pregnancy, labour and birth are a miraculous cocktail and a very complex subject. We do not need to go into the details for our purposes, but we will take a simple look. When we are in the emergency response – when the sympathetic nervous system is activated – we produce hormones called catecholamines and in particular adrenaline, which is the most important hormone from our point of view. We all know what an adrenaline rush feels like. Maybe you have been driving down a road when a car shoots out in front of you. You jam your foot on the brake and it feels almost like an electric shock shooting down your back. Your heart starts to thump, pumping blood around your body in case you need to run or fight. And your eyes are out on stalks panning for predators, because if there has been one sabre-toothed tiger there might be another.

All your resources, all your energy, go to your arms and your legs, ready to run or fight – which is a great system for dealing with sabre-toothed tigers but absolutely useless when you're in labour, because you are not going anywhere.

That's how the sympathetic nervous system works.

The confident response – the parasympathetic nervous system

The other system that controls our responses is the parasympathetic nervous system. This is the state we are in most of the time because most of the time is not an emergency. The two systems cannot function at the same time. You may be feeling fine as you read this book, so your parasympathetic nervous system is functioning, and you feel confident and relaxed. When we are in the confident response – when the parasympathetic nervous system is activated – we produce the hormone oxytocin (again looking somewhat simplistically at this complex system). Oxytocin has been described by the Swedish scientist Kerstin Uvnäs-Moberg as the hormone of 'calmness and co-operation'. Michel Odent, the French obstetrician and natural birth pioneer, calls it the hormone of love, because we produce great peaks of it at special times in our lives. We produce bursts of it when we fall in love and when we make love, and the biggest peak of all is the one a mother produces just after she has given birth. It promotes the bonding of mother and baby and the establishment of breastfeeding.

We love the feeling oxytocin gives us; we are addicted to it and would do practically anything for a fix. It is probably the hormone that has ensured the continuation of the human race. Oxytocin is also the hormone that makes the uterine muscles work in labour. Therefore, as long as you are feeling confident, calm and harmonious, you will naturally produce this hormone which makes the uterine muscles work and makes labour efficient.

Another important hormone we produce in the parasympathetic nervous system, or the confidence response, is endorphins. Endorphins, as their full name 'endogenous morphine' implies, are related to morphine. Morphine is the most powerful pain-relieving artificial drug that we have. We give it to people after major surgery and with advanced cancer. Endorphins, which we produce naturally in our own bodies, have been said to be many times more powerful than morphine. In her book *The Oxytocin Factor*, Kerstin Uvnäs-Moberg says that when we feel calm and confident, the elevated level of oxytocin in the body seems to result in the increased secretion of endorphins. So if the mind is in the right place, the body naturally produces oxytocin to make labour efficient, and endorphins to make it comfortable.

When a mother is in the parasympathetic nervous system, all her resources, all her blood supply and oxygen, go to her internal organs − to her digestive system so she can digest food to keep her energy up in labour, and to her reproductive organs. This is a far more efficient use of energy than diverting it to the arms and legs, as with the fear response.

The system is perfect, and already in place. It is very simple: the most beautiful shining diamond.

The trouble is that we tend to get in the way, and hypnobirthing is the system that helps us to let go of the thoughts which get in the way of this perfect system and allow it to work well.

What is it that trips us from the parasympathetic nervous system, the confident response, to the sympathetic nervous system, the emergency response? It is two things – fear, and being observed. It is why many people are petrified of public speaking. It is totally unnatural for any animal to stand out in the open and be observed. They skulk in the undergrowth, or seek safety in numbers in a herd, or they are camouflaged against their background like a camel in the desert. It's also why labour frequently slows down when a mother arrives at a birth centre or hospital. However friendly the environment and kind the midwives, she is still in a strange place being observed by strange people, and the natural response of her body is to freeze. It doesn't have to be abject terror; it is simply a very subtle, animal suspicion.

You cannot be in both the sympathetic and the parasympathetic nervous systems at the same time. You cannot be in the fear response and the confident response.

Let's just recap what we have looked at.

The body is designed to produce oxytocin, which makes birth efficient, and endorphins, which make birth comfortable, as long as our minds are in a calm, safe and harmonious place. Therefore labour will be efficient and labour will be comfortable.

The system is perfect; it is already in place.

All we need to do is let go of the fears and the worries and the negative thoughts that we have all acquired about birth.

This is why hypnobirthing works so very well. Every time you practise hypnobirthing techniques you are letting go, you are releasing – allowing your body to give birth naturally, comfortably and easily.

CHAPTER 3

The Mind/Body Effect

'Giving birth can be the most
empowering experience of a lifetime –
an initiation into a new dimension
of mind-body awareness.'

Ina May Gaskin,
Birth Matters, 2011

The Mind/Body Effect

Let us now consider the power of the mind. Everybody accepts that the thoughts in your mind affect your body. If somebody is feeling depressed you can instantly see it in the way they walk. If you have to tell someone bad news, you suggest that they sit down first in case they feel weak at the knees. But we sometimes underestimate just how powerful the mind is. We tend to assume that everything happens in the body, and that the mind merely has some effect on what goes on.

W hen you think about it, the body is merely a hunk of meat. It does absolutely nothing without the mind telling it to. So effectively, everything happens in the mind, and the body just trots dutifully along behind and does what it is told.

I'd like you to do a little exercise with each other as a couple, or with a friend.

Stand opposite each other, and mothers, stretch out an arm in front of you and put your hand palm upwards on your partner's shoulder, keeping your arm straight. Make sure the palm is facing up, otherwise you can twist your elbow. Now fathers, try to bend her arm downwards at the elbow and

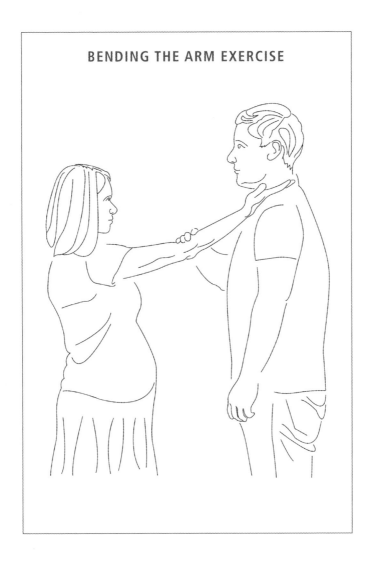

BENDING THE ARM EXERCISE

mothers, try to resist him with all your strength. Now, given that a man is stronger than a woman, her arm will probably bend, though you may be surprised how strong she is.

Just relax for a minute, mothers shake your arm out, then put your arm back onto his shoulder in a very relaxed way. This time remain relaxed, and focus your attention on the tips of your fingers or even beyond, maybe looking towards a picture on the wall, or out of the window. You could imagine that someone has drawn a picture of flowers of different colours on your fingertips – but whatever you choose, focus your attention very firmly on the tips of your fingers or beyond.

Now fathers, try once more to bend her arm. Do it gently to start with because she has not done this exercise before, and help her to keep her attention right out in front of her, but build up the pressure on the arm gradually. And mothers, you may well find that, as long as your focus stays out there, the arm is much stronger than it was before. It also feels much easier to keep a straight arm than when you were resisting only with physical strength the first time. Interesting! Practise this a few times because, as with everything, we get better with practice.

The arm exercise shows us that if we relax our body and focus our mind, our body can work more efficiently and more comfortably than when we use only our physical strength. This knowledge applies not just to the arm exercise but also to the body in labour. By doing the exercise you will know and have felt this for yourself.

Up breathing

There are two types of breathing in hypnobirthing. The first we'll learn is the breathing that you will use during surges in the Up stage (first stage) of labour. It is also the breathing you use during practice. Because the muscles are drawing up during a surge, I call it the 'up breathing', and it is very simple. It is a long, slow breath, in through the nose and out through the mouth.

The purpose of this breath is to use the absolute minimum of muscular effort, so that the muscles used in breathing in no way inhibit the working of the uterine muscles. We breathe in through the nose because it is a natural way of breathing; we breathe out through the mouth because that gives a feeling of release – it's a letting go, and that is exactly what we want to achieve. Even something as simple as a few slow, deep breaths can help you feel more relaxed and completely change the atmosphere around you. Try that now and you'll see that it's true.

I would suggest to start with that you count quickly and breathe in for a count of 15 and out for a count of 20. For some people this may be too long, so please adapt the count to what is right for you. You may, for example, want to do 12 in and 15 out – and I stress again this is a quick count. If you're a flautist or a singer you can probably count 30 in and 40 out perfectly easily. But the really important thing is that you're not straining to achieve a particular breath, that it is entirely relaxed, and you are not holding to achieve any particular length of count. Of course, as you practise it will become more natural and the breaths will gradually lengthen.

The length of breath you can achieve also depends upon the stage of pregnancy you are at because, as your baby grows, your lung capacity is increasingly reduced. And then suddenly, in the last couple of weeks before birth, the baby's head engages in your pelvis, your baby moves down, and you can breathe more easily. All these factors make a difference.

Practise this now. Count quickly through one breath and see how it feels, breathing in through the nose and out through the mouth. Let the air flow out and then breathe in – 2, 3, 4, 5, 6, 7, 8, 9, 10, 11, 12, 13, 14, 15, and out – 2, 3, 4, 5, 6, 7, 8, 9, 10, 11, 12, 13, 14, 15, 16, 17, 18, 19, 20. You can make it shorter or longer if you want, but this is about right for most people. Now do the same again, but this time do three breaths, because three or four breaths are more like the length of a surge.

We know that the uterine muscles are working to draw up, and we know that the mind is powerful and affects the body. We have just done an exercise to prove it. Therefore, if the body is working upwards, we want the mind to be thinking 'up' so that mind and body are working together. So there are some visualisations to go with this breathing.

One visualisation you might find useful is to imagine the sun rising, because as the sun comes up, that lovely pink appears on the horizon and may be reflected in the clouds above. Visualise the sun coming up as you breathe in, and as you exhale, see it rising higher and higher in the sky as it does during the morning. Another helpful visualisation is, as you breathe in, to see yourself blowing bubbles that get bigger and bigger. Then as you breathe out, the bubbles just dance gently upwards into the sky.

Practise the up breathing exercise with these visualisations. It's ideal to have someone to talk you through the visualisations, and they can use the suggestions that follow, but you can practise on your own as well, and you will soon remember the images.

It's much easier to visualise with your eyes closed, so you are not distracted by whatever is going on around you. So, allow your eyes to gently close, count for one breath as you did before – counting in for 15, out for 20 – and then on the next breath watch the sun rise, the beautiful pink appearing on the horizon, and as you breathe out, breathe up with the sun as it rises higher in the sky.

On the next breath, see yourself blowing bubbles, see them getting bigger and bigger, and as you breathe out watch the bubbles float away upwards into the sky. Take one more breath, and as you breathe in, notice that with each upward breath your body becomes more relaxed and calm, and as you exhale, breathe up as your mind and body work together in unison.

UP-BREATHING VISUALISATIONS

Watch the sun rise, the beautiful pink appearing on the horizon.

Breathe up with the sun as it rises higher in the sky.

As the sun rises, so your body draws gently upwards.

See yourself blowing bubbles, and see them get bigger and bigger.

Watch the bubbles float upwards into the sky, upwards into the sky, drawing upwards with each relaxing breath.

Breathe slowly, and very comfortably.

With each soothing breath your body becomes more relaxed and calm.

Breathe up as your mind and body work together in unison.

You're doing really well; that's very good.

So calm, so serene, so at peace.

These visualisations may be helpful, but you can use anything that is comforting and relaxing for you and has an 'up' emphasis. You may find it helpful if your birth companion prompts you with these suggestions during surges. Fathers are welcome to use their own words, but if they have been up all night they may not be at their most creative at 3am, so it can be useful to have some suggestions ready. They can say the same thing over and over again, which is quite soothing, like a mantra. Or they can say something very simple like, 'You're doing really well and I love you.' And some women prefer silence.

Even something as simple as relaxed breathing gets better with practice. So I would suggest that you practise this slow breathing together with the visualisations a couple of times a day. For many couples, the best times of the day can be first thing in the morning and last thing at night, because then you are both together. It is a great excuse for not leaping out of bed as soon as you wake up! However, if this is your second baby, first thing in the morning is probably not a peaceful time, so it might be when you come home from work, or another time that works for you. Take just two or three minutes to practise the breathing using visualisations just as you have done now, so that it becomes second nature.

The up breathing is what you will use during surges in the up stage of labour, and also for practising relaxations beforehand. Use it now for the following exercise.

Find someone to read this script for you, slowly and quietly, perhaps with some gentle music in the background. The music I use for practice and which is also ideal to play while your baby is being born is the CD *River Dawn: Piano Meditations*, composed and played by Catherine Marie Charlton. It is music played on a real piano by a real person, rather than electronic music, which has a completely different effect. Catherine Marie composed it for use with hypnotherapy, and she used it with the relaxations in this book for the birth of her own baby. Fathers can read the script for mothers, and then swap over, so that you can both experience it.

COTTAGE SUPPER

Let the air flow out and breathe in – 2, 3, 4, 5, 6, 7, 8, 9, 10, 11, 12, 13, 14, 15, and out – 2, 3, 4, 5, 6, 7, 8, 9, 10, 11, 12, 13, 14, 15, 16, 17, 18, 19, 20. If you gently close your eyes, it's easier to notice sounds. Just for a minute or two, listen to the sound of your breathing as it becomes longer ... slower ... deeper ... Now, as the breath drifts down inside you and brings serenity and relaxation throughout your body, begin to observe the sound of the chatter in your head. As you listen quietly, notice that it gradually softens, and fades into oblivion. Now rest your attention on the sounds in the room and, as they fade, hear the silence. Allow your attention to expand to the whole building, hear the silence, the street, the city – now include the whole country. Allow the silence to wash over you, wider and wider, until it encompasses the whole world, out and out, further and further, deeper and deeper silence.

Now visualise yourself coming to the end of a long walk. It's been a wonderful day, but you've been walking for many miles and you're tired now. You had a picnic at lunchtime, but that was hours ago, and now you're ravenously hungry. You wonder what's for dinner.

As you approach the friendly, welcoming cottage where you are staying, you notice the garden gate in front of you. Notice what colour it is. Notice the material it's made of. Now put out your hand and touch it, notice if it is warm or cold, smooth or rough. As you open the gate, feel its weight on the hinges, and hear the sound of the hinges as it swings open.

Continued overleaf...

... *Continued from page 47*

As you walk into the garden, feel the texture of the path beneath your feet, and hear the sound of your footfalls on the path. This garden is full of beautiful, colourful flowers, and you stop to smell a voluptuous and beautiful rose. Feel the velvety softness of the petals on your cheeks; notice the delicate scent. Hear the hum of bees as they collect the pollen; feel the warmth of the last rays of the setting sun. In the distance, the first owl hoots softly.

As you open the door of the cottage, you notice that someone has been baking, as the enticing smell lingers in the little hallway. Is it a delicious cake, or freshly baked bread? Notice the changes taking place in your mouth. You open the kitchen door, and the much stronger aroma of supper fills your nostrils. Your mind fills with images of the delicious, freshly made meal that has been lovingly prepared for you, and you sit down at the table ready to start eating.

Now open your eyes. What happened then?

Many people find that they salivate. You may have, you may not have. If I tell you to salivate you can't do it on command; it's an involuntary response. But the ideas that you put in your head can make you salivate, just like Pavlov's dogs. It's just the same with labour. Labour is an involuntary response, but the ideas that you put in your head can affect its progress and its comfort.

Not everybody will salivate during the above exercise. Most people do, but a few don't because everybody is different – we all respond to different things and learn in different ways.

For example, some people are visual learners, who learn from seeing how things are done, while others are more auditory and prefer to be talked through things. That's why you are given many different things to practise in hypnobirthing. You don't have to do them all, but simply choose those you like best. This is good to know, because people sometimes have a fear that hypnotherapy can make you do or say something you would rather not — which is completely impossible, because nobody can use hypnotherapy to make you do something when you don't want to, or that is not in your best interests.

I'm sure you know the colour of the rose that you smelt during the exercise — maybe it was pink or red, or white or yellow. And when you were thinking about the place you were staying, it was as if you were actually there, and you forgot the place where you are sitting now. The cottage setting was much more real than what's going on for you at this moment. It's just a little exercise, but very useful.

Down breathing

The first type of breathing we have learnt involves drawing upwards during the first or up stage of labour: as the muscles draw up, the walls of the uterus thin and the cervix opens. We do what I call the 'down breathing' once the cervix is fully opened, as the baby moves down the birth passage into the world. Let's practise this now. It is a quick breath in through the nose, and a longer breath out through the nose. There is no particular count to it.

The reason for breathing out through the nose this time is that it is a much more focused breathing. It is almost as if your breath is following the baby down; you can practically feel it on the pelvic floor focusing downwards — not forcing downwards, focusing downwards. Try it for yourself a few times: a short breath in through the nose and a longer breath out through the nose, focusing your attention downwards.

Just like the up breathing, there are visualisations to go with the down breathing. An image of anything that is down, soft and open can be helpful. You can try visualising the ripples going out on a pond where a fish has risen; the ripples move out and out and out, so fluid and soft, smoother and smoother. It's a lovely visualisation.

Or it can be helpful to imagine a full-blown rose, or any flower you like. It feels so soft and velvety on your cheeks as you inhale its sweet fragrance. It is a soft and open image, and if your mind is thinking soft and open, your body is doing soft and open. You may have seen a speeded-up image of a flower opening, and imagining something like that can be very helpful.

Another helpful image is of a little waterfall. If you go for a walk in the mountains and finding a stream trickling down into a small waterfall, you could sit there entranced for hours, watching the sunshine glinting on the drops of water. Any soft and open or 'downwards' images like this are very helpful and effective.

You can use the prompts on the opposite page while you do the down breathing, or better still, your husband or partner can read them for you.

Take a few minutes to practise the down breathing with the visualisations. Take a quick breath in, and as you breathe out imagine that full-blown flower, beautiful, soft, velvety and voluptuous. Breathe in, and breathing out see the ripples going out on the pond, fluid, soft and open. One more, breathe in, and as you breathe out imagine that delightful little mountain waterfall. You can sit there entranced watching the sunshine on the drops of water, downwards, soft and gentle.

As with the visualisations for the up breathing, keep it simple. For both stages I have given you lots of examples, but

DOWN-BREATHING VISUALISATIONS

Imagine a beautiful full-blown rose, so soft and velvety and open.

Watch the ripples flowing out and out on a pond. Fluid and smooth and open.

Your body eases your baby gently down with each breath.

Imagine an entrancing waterfall, with the water flowing gently downwards.

Trust the gentle downward movement of your body and your baby.

Your baby moves easily downwards.

With each breath, your baby is coming to you.

Focus your attention down towards your baby.

You will soon be holding your baby in your arms.

you might find that you prefer just to say the same thing over and over again, like a mantra. The phrases I have given are only suggestions, but at three in the morning when you're not at your best, they can be useful to have at hand. And if your husband or partner is reading for you and you would find a different image more helpful, then he can change to something else. But, fathers, you can say whatever you like, or keep it really simple. Saying something as simple as

'You're doing really well and I love you,' is more than adequate. Use the examples as guidelines which you may find useful during labour.

Please practise the down breathing. Have your husband or partner read aloud so that you can practise the visualisations, and it all becomes intuitive ready for when your baby is born. Many women have said they couldn't have done it without him, and it was his voice that carried them through.

Practise on the loo as well. Sometimes in late pregnancy you can get a little constipated. After all, there is a head in your pelvis! Practising the down breathing on the loo proves to you that it works even before you have your baby. It is multi-tasking – very efficient.

CHAPTER 4

Preparing Your Baby and Body For Birth

'In an ideal world, the main preoccupation of doctors and other health professionals involved in pre-natal care should be to protect the emotional state of pregnant women.'

Michel Odent,
The Caesarean, 2004

Preparing Your Baby and Body For Birth

You have probably come to hypnobirthing to help you achieve a more comfortable birth. Most of the work of hypnobirthing is done in the practice before your baby's birth. This chapter covers other simple suggestions which you can use together with hypnobirthing to help you achieve the birth you want.

O n the opposite page is a picture of a baby in the perfect position ready for birth. I would like you to photocopy it and put it up somewhere in your home where you will see it frequently, such as on the fridge, by your bed, or perhaps opposite the loo, and make a point of noticing the image as you pass it because what we put in our mind affects our body, as we have seen in the previous chapter. Just notice this picture every time you pass it.

Back-to-back babies

Most babies move into the position shown in the picture in late pregnancy. The baby's head is down and facing to your right, and during labour the baby turns to face your back. However, some babies face the front, with their back against yours: a back–to–back baby. We heard about one in Chapter 1.

The heaviest part of the head is at the occiput, which is the bone at the base of the skull. By virtue of gravity, the

THE MOST USUAL POSITION READY FOR BIRTH

My baby is in the best position for a calm
and natural birth.

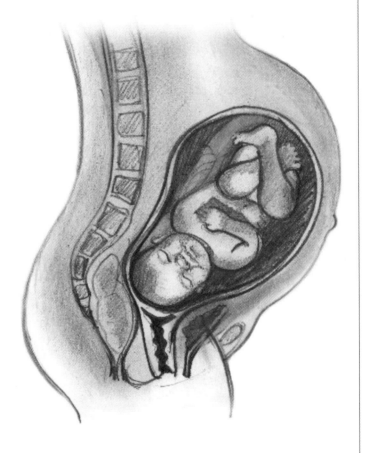

My body and my baby's body work
together in unison.

heaviest part will always go to the lowest point. So, in our modern world, if a pregnant mother comes home from work and flops down on the sofa, the lowest point is her back and therefore the heaviest part of the baby's head (the occiput) will be encouraged to go towards her back and so the baby faces the front. If you have your car seat sloping backwards, then when you joggle as you drive, the back of the baby's head is encouraged to go towards your back. It is thought that possibly there are more back-to-back babies than there used to be as a result of our modern lifestyle, because in previous ages people would have been more upright.

Poor people would only have had wooden chairs. If you visit a stately home, you will find that the chairs there are much more upright than today's. You can imagine people sitting on them sewing or reading, not flopping in front of the television. People would also have spent more time scrubbing floors, working in the fields, digging in the garden; all things where you lean forwards. If you wanted to get somewhere, most people would have walked, and so you would have been leaning slightly forwards joggling your baby. Babies would have been much more encouraged to have the back of their heads towards the front.

Preparing your body

From now until your baby is born, it's a very good idea to be in a more upright position. Birthing balls are wonderful things to sit on. They are just big gym balls, and the idea is that when you sit on the ball your hips should be slightly higher than your knees. You can get birthing balls in several sizes and blow them up appropriately. They can be used at your desk when you are working, or to sit at the table when you are having a meal. Because they are round you tend to move slightly, which flexes your back and helps it to stay supple and comfortable. They can also be very comfortable to sit on during labour.

If you commute to work, maybe you could get off the train or bus one stop early and walk a little way, because walking will encourage your baby to be in the more usual position facing your back.

When sitting on the sofa, instead of flopping backwards, you could sit cross-legged and propped up on cushions. Not only is it more upright, but sitting cross-legged tends to stretch the tissue of the inner thighs and the pelvic floor, which is the tissue that will stretch during labour. And if you want a bigger stretch, instead of sitting with your legs crossed, sit in the same position but with the soles of your feet together and you will feel the stretch in your inner thighs. The more you bring your feet towards you, the more the tissue stretches, and by gently bouncing your knees the stretch is even more effective, so the muscle tissue becomes even more elastic. As we know, elastic not only stretches but springs back again afterwards – both very good when you are having a baby. But please avoid this stretching exercise if your midwife or obstetrician advise against it.

Squatting

Another good and very natural position is squatting. If you put a toy in the centre of the floor and brought in a two-year-old, the child would run in and squat down to play with it – they wouldn't sit or kneel or stand; they would squat. There are many societies around the world where people squat in a circle and chat to their friends all evening. It's very comfortable.

The trouble is that when we first went to school, we thought it was awfully sophisticated to sit on chairs, and we lost the knack of squatting. I would suggest that squatting is

THE SQUATTING POSITION

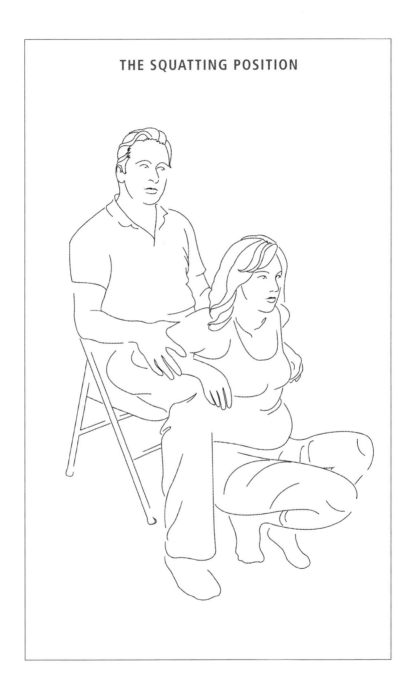

a good thing to practise during pregnancy. You don't need to practise for hours each day, but maybe when you settle to watch your favourite television programme, instead of sitting on the sofa, squat in front of it with your elbows resting on it behind you for support. The only problem we have with squatting is that it feels rather wobbly to start with. Just do it for five minutes to begin with, and you'll probably find that it is a very comfortable position. At the end of the week you may find yourself still squatting there half an hour later at the end of the programme.

A particularly comfortable way of squatting when you give birth is squatting between your husband's or your partner's legs as he sits on a chair behind you. You can support yourself on his legs, you have human warmth all around you, and he can gently massage your back and whisper prompts in your ear. It's a very comfortable position for giving birth – if you feel like it.

There is a great deal of talk about the best position for giving birth, and there are books with many very complicated pictures. But consider, if you were going for a walk in the country and wanted to open your bowels, you would retire behind a tree, and you wouldn't stand there considering what position to take, you would just squat, because it's the natural way to expel anything from your body. It's exactly the same having a baby: your body knows what to do. But if it's your first baby, your brain doesn't yet know that your body can do it perfectly well. In the event, you will simply go into whatever position is comfortable for you and will help your baby most.

As you squat down you can almost feel your hips easing outwards, and the capacity of your pelvis can be up to 30 per cent greater compared with lying on your back (according to X-ray studies on 'primitive' upright delivery positions by J.G.B. Russell in the 1980s).

It is said that women only began to give birth lying on their backs in the time of Louis XIV, because the king expressed a wish to see a baby being born when his mistress was giving birth. At that time women in labour would often sit on stools, such as milking stools, and the midwife would receive the baby at floor level; but kings don't grovel on the floor, so it all had to be frightfully proper and his mistress lay in bed. Women of the court copied this, and midwives began to find they had more difficulty getting babies out when the mothers lay flat, so they called in the doctors more often. Then everyone started giving birth lying down, believing that if it was done in the royal household, it must be best – but nobody quite thought about what was actually best for the mother and the baby.

Squatting is one of the best and most natural positions for childbirth. You have gravity on your side and you have the maximum pelvic capacity. It shortens the length of the birth passage and helps your baby to move more quickly and easily into the world. It also tilts the uterus and pelvis forward, placing the baby in the proper alignment for birth, and opens the pelvic floor muscles. So do practise squatting for a few minutes each day and then it will be an option which feels natural and will be there for you if you choose to give birth in this position.

If you give birth lying flat or nearly flat, not only do you not have gravity on your side but, because of the curl of the coccyx, you are actually pushing upwards, which is pushing against gravity. As the baby moves down towards birth, the coccyx naturally flexes and moves out of the way. But if you are lying flat on your back it can't do that, because your weight and the bed are preventing it, and therefore you are making the space your baby has to come through smaller.

A mother is often most comfortable giving birth in an upright position, probably leaning slightly forwards, squatting, kneeling, leaning on the kitchen work surface, or standing up with her arms around her husband's or her partner's neck – so that the weight of her body in no way inhibits her blood flow or her nervous system. But always consider your individual circumstances – there is no 'one size fits all'. If, for instance, a woman has pelvic girdle pain in pregnancy, squatting may not be appropriate for her, and it might be wise to seek medical advice and consider getting any lumbar or sacral misalignments corrected by a craniosacral therapist or a McTimoney chiropractor before giving birth.

Breech babies

Remember also that some babies are not positioned with their head down – these are breech babies, with their bottom down instead. Some babies can be lying across the womb or at an oblique angle – a transverse baby. If a baby is genuinely transverse when you go into labour, neither its head nor its buttocks are positioned to move into the birth passage ready for birth, and you can be grateful that a Caesarean section is available. But if your baby is transverse towards the end of pregnancy, it could be that it is in the process of turning to the head down position ready for birth. Most babies will turn from whatever they're happily doing before to a head-down position between about week 30 and week 35 to 37 of pregnancy. So if anybody tells you that your baby is breech at 32 weeks, it isn't. It just hasn't turned yet. About a third of babies are in a breech position at 28 weeks but only three or four in a hundred are still breech at 40 weeks.

There may be perfectly good reasons why the baby has decided to be breech. We're out here, he or she is inside, and it seems very presumptuous to think that we necessarily know better. We do know that it may be easier for a baby to be born head down and facing the mother's back. But the baby may be breech due to the position of the umbilical cord, the position of the placenta, or the shape of the uterus, in which case breech could be the best position for that baby. The phrase 'baby knows best' is one we would do well to consider seriously in many circumstances. On the other hand, it may be breech simply because it never got round to turning and space became limited as it grew and turning became harder, in which case some encouragement might help the baby to turn.

There are various ways of helping a breech baby to turn, and the one that you will be offered is an ECV – an External Cephalic Version – at about 37 weeks. An ECV is a powerful manipulation to turn the baby from the outside, using very firm touch on your baby through your tummy, which can be uncomfortable. The risk of an ECV is that, as the baby is manipulated round and pressure is put on the baby to turn, it could pull the cord and therefore the placenta. If the placenta starts to bleed you would need a Caesarean section straight away. So you don't want an ECV to be too early and you don't want it to be too late. ECVs are up to 50 per cent successful; you may want to ask the person who is going to do it what their success rate is, as there are quite big variations.

There are techniques that may help a breech baby to turn. You can rub the points used in acupuncture for yourself. Acupressure has been said to be an older art than acupuncture. The story goes that it became known in ancient China that various points on the body could be massaged to encourage and maintain health. This system became widely known, and came to the ears of the emperor, so the best practitioner was called in to treat him. But then there was a problem because ordinary people were not allowed to touch the emperor, so a system of using needles was devised instead. If the emperor was treated with needles, it obviously had to be best, so the use of needles became universal. I have absolutely no idea if there is any truth in this, or if it is just a delightful story.

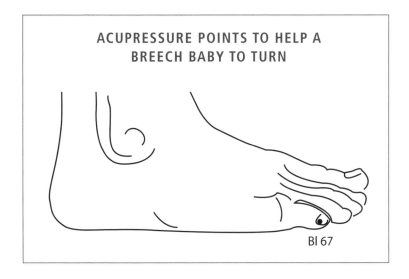

Take a line along the outside of your foot from your heel to your little toe and massage vigorously the point where that line reaches the outside corner of the bed of your little toe nail on both feet. The precise point is called Bladder 67 (Bl 67) – see the illustration above. For professional advice on this, make an appointment with an acupuncturist.

The homoeopathic remedy frequently used is pulsatilla; a homeopath can give you informed advice on this.

Some people have put an ice pack on the top of the abdomen and shone a light and played gentle music at the lower end of the abdomen to persuade a breech baby that being head down may be a more comfortable position.

But in her book *Breech Birth*, Benna Waites quotes research from Dr Mehl's study in 1994 which found that hypnotherapy had an 81 per cent success rate and was the most effective way of turning a breech baby. When I work with a mother and her breech baby, it never ceases to amaze me how effective hypnotherapy is. I have no idea if I am talking to the mother or to the baby, or simply relaxing the mother so that it's easy for the baby to turn. I know how important it is to say all the right things, but I leave thinking, 'It's only me talking. How can that possibly make a difference?' But 80 per cent of the time, the next morning I get a call saying, 'The baby turned.'

We spoke earlier about the power of words, so talk to your breech baby. Acknowledge that your baby might be in the right position, because of the shape of the uterus, or the position of the cord or the placenta. But suggest that it might like to turn and that it could be more comfortable for it, while still acknowledging that your baby may well have got it right. So often, baby knows best.

Squatting is not a good idea if you have gone to about 35 weeks and you know your baby is breech, because as you squat you open the pelvis and encourage the baby down into it. If the baby's head is downwards, that is thoroughly beneficial. If it is not, don't squat until the baby turns head down, and then squat as much as you like to encourage the head to move well down into the pelvis. However, swimming can be good to encourage your baby to float into a different position. Remember that only about 4 per cent of babies are still in a breech presentation at the end of pregnancy, so it's not very likely to happen, and your baby can turn at any time – at week 39, and even occasionally in labour.

There was a trial in 2001 called the Hannah Trial, which compared Caesarean sections for breech babies with assisted deliveries by an obstetrician. Those running the trial said the outcome suggested that a Caesarean section was safer than an assisted vaginal delivery, and from that point on all breech babies started to be delivered by Caesarean. Since then, the methodology of the trial has been brought into question and there is a strong body of opinion among midwives and parents that it is safer for a breech baby to be born vaginally with a natural birth under the care of a midwife, than for the mother to have elective major abdominal surgery before it is known whether the baby can and will be born smoothly in breech position.

Because of the policy of delivering breech babies by Caesarean section, midwives and doctors have less experience in delivering breech babies. Some hospitals are beginning to change their policy to support normal breech births, with Canada and France leading the way in this work, and there are a few early signs that this practice is beginning to be adopted in the UK. A breech baby has been described as 'normal but unusual' by Mary Cronk, the midwife who probably has more experience attending mothers giving birth to a breech baby than anyone in the UK, so it can be a perfectly sensible option to give birth to your baby vaginally, naturally and normally, if you can be attended by somebody with the experience and skill to assist you.

I have known mothers whose breech babies have turned, and I have known mothers who have given birth to a breech baby completely normally with a natural vaginal birth. So you do have options and, should you find yourself in that situation, do some more research. I strongly recommend you look at the booklet 'Breech Birth: What Are My Options?', published by an organisation called AIMS (Association for Improvements in the Maternity Services). They produce many good booklets which you can get from their website, www.aims.org.uk. There are more details about AIMS at the back of this book.

If you would like an objective second opinion on this or any other medical matter, consult an independent midwife.

Pelvic floor exercises

People go on about pelvic floor exercises ad nauseam and the trouble is they are incredibly boring. You probably forget to do them and then go to sleep at night resolving to do them tomorrow; but then the next day exactly the same thing happens.

Pelvic floor exercises are useful for two reasons: you *tense* the muscles of the pelvic floor, starting at the back passage, moving forwards and right up into the vagina, hold it for a few seconds, and then *release*. The tensing is important because it tones muscles, and toned muscles work better. The releasing is also important because you are programming yourself to let go when you feel tension – so as you feel the pressure of your baby's head passing down the birth passage, you let go, and the baby's journey into the world is easier for both of you. For both reasons, pelvic floor exercises are good, so make them easy for yourself.

Make them habitual so that they happen automatically during 'down time' in your life, because we all have down time every day. Most of us sit in front of a computer screen cursing that it is so slow booting up or downloading something. We can use that time to do pelvic floor exercises. You can put a little note on the screen that says 'Pelvic Floor Exercises' or 'PFE', which will mean nothing to anyone but you. One father said he was going to send his wife an email every day saying 'Pelvic Floor Exercises' – which is a good idea, but it would be even better to send a large attachment with it that takes a long time to download.

Another time you might like to do them is if you're on the bus or the train going into work, or in the car at red traffic lights. When the traffic lights go red there's almost always time for a couple of pelvic floor exercises before they go green again. Everybody has some down time that offers the perfect chance to practise pelvic floor exercises, and after a few times you will have programmed yourself so that, for example, if you see a red traffic light you automatically do your pelvic floor exercises without having to make a conscious effort to remember. In hypnotherapy terms it's called an 'anchor', and so that stimulus is an anchor for pelvic floor exercises to happen. You don't have to think about it and remember it any more. It just happens.

Pelvic floor exercises are a very useful preparation for the birth of your baby, and they are also an efficient way of helping your body get back to normal after the birth. Once you have programmed yourself to do them, it is a useful training for the whole of your life.

Perineal massage

Massaging your perineum (the area between the vagina and the anus) and the vagina with oil softens the tissue and makes it more elastic. It makes sense, because soft tissue is more flexible. We put face cream on our face and put hand cream on our hands to soften the tissue, so we have already bought into the idea that we can make a difference to the flexibility of our bodies, and so it makes sense to prepare the vagina and pelvic floor ready for birth. Elastic, as we know, 'gives' easily and also springs back easily afterwards.

Research into perineal massage found that expectant mothers who massage the perineum, from week 34 of pregnancy, reduce the likelihood of tearing and the need for an episiotomy (when the perineum is surgically cut to help the baby's delivery).

By massaging the perineum like this once a day, you will notice the area becoming more flexible and you will become more used to feeling the stretching sensations that also occur during birth.

It does make sense; it does make a difference. If perineal massage doesn't appeal to you, weigh this up against the possibility of tearing and stitches when you have your baby, and there is really no competition. All these things add up to a more comfortable birth.

HOW TO DO PERINEAL MASSAGE

- **Wash your hands** thoroughly.

- **Sit or lie back** in a private, warm and comfortable place.

- **Apply a lubricant** such as olive oil, baby massage oil or sweet almond oil (or any neutral oil) to your hands and the perineal area.

- **Place both thumbs** about 3cm into the vagina.

- **Massage the area** by gently rubbing the perineal tissues between your thumbs and fingers.

- **Press downwards** and to the sides, gently stretching until you feel a tingling sensation.

- **Once this sensation** is felt, hold the stretch for around one minute until the feeling subsides, and begin gently massaging the lower part of the vagina by moving your thumbs back and forth. While massaging also hook your thumbs on the sides of the vagina and gently pull the tissue forwards, as your baby's head does when it is being born.

- **Continue to gently rub** *as you stretch, for around three to four minutes.*

CHAPTER 5

Nutrition

'Let food be your medicine.'

Hippocrates, *c.* 400 BC

Nutrition

You would never dream of putting the wrong fuel in your car. It would break down. But many of us consistently put the wrong fuel in our bodies, which are such amazing self-healing machines that they continue working for years until ultimately something has to give – a large contributory factor to the chronic diseases of old age.

W hen you become pregnant, you suddenly become more aware of what you put in your body because it will affect your baby. If you are wise, both you and your partner will have been taking extra care for months before you became pregnant, in order that both your bodies were in the best possible state of health when your baby was conceived. As a result, you are probably feeling a great deal healthier and more energetic, so you already realise the difference good nutrition makes. Here are a few guidelines.

Water

Our bodies are made up of between 50 and 70 per cent water so we need to maintain our intake of water for good health. Neither our brain nor our body functions at its best if we are dehydrated. Drinking alcohol depletes the water in the body. Drinking plenty of water (I mean plain water, not some other substance mixed with water) helps to keep us free from morning sickness and prevent pre-eclampsia. If you already have morning sickness, adding a squeeze of lemon or a teaspoon of cider vinegar to the water, or drinking it at room temperature, can be helpful.

Diet

Do

If you are already eating healthily, you can simply continue to do so and it is very likely you will feel healthy and well throughout your pregnancy. The greatest deficiency in our diet is often vegetables. We are told we should have the famous 'five a day' of fruit and vegetables so we reach for the fruit bowl as we rush past. Aim for five a day of vegetables (not the high glycaemic index vegetables like carrots and potatoes, though these can be included in moderation) and top up with fruit occasionally. Our modern diet tends to be too acidifying, and a greater emphasis on alkalising foods can have a beneficial impact on our health. To help you, here are some alkalising and acidifying foods:

Some alkalising foods

Almonds, apples, apricots, avocados, bananas, beans, beetroot, blackberries, broccoli, Brussels sprouts, cabbage, carrots, cauliflower, celery, chard, cherries, coconut, cucumbers, dates (dried), dried fruit, figs, goat's milk, grapefruit, grapes, green beans, green peas, lemon, lettuce, melon, millet, mushrooms, onions, oranges, parsnips, peaches, pears, pineapple, potatoes, radishes, raisins, raspberries, rhubarb, root vegetables, sauerkraut, spinach, strawberries, tangerines, tomatoes, watercress, watermelon.

Some acidifying foods

Bacon, beef, blueberries, bran, brazil nuts, butter, cheese, chicken, cod, corn, corned beef, cow's milk, crackers, cranberries, currants, eggs, fish, haddock, herrings, lamb, lentils (dried), mackerel, mayonnaise, macaroni, oats, olives, peanut butter, peanuts, peas (dried), plums, pork, prunes, rice, rye, salmon, sardines, sausages, shellfish, spaghetti, sunflower seeds, turkey, walnuts, wheat, yoghurt.

I am not suggesting that you should suddenly become vegetarian. Indeed, meat and oily fish are thoroughly beneficial in pregnancy because your baby needs protein and essential fatty acids in order to grow, but you might consider a shift of emphasis as you become more aware of your health for the sake of your baby.

Protein is important for your developing baby. The amino acids that make up protein form the building blocks of your, and your baby's body cells. If you are vegetarian, quinoa, said to be almost the perfect food, is probably the best source of protein you can have. It contains more protein than a grain, more essential fatty acids than fruit, and is rich in calcium, iron, B vitamins and vitamin E. It is low in fat, and the essential fatty acids support the development of your baby's nervous system and brain. Even if you are not vegetarian, flaked quinoa added to your breakfast cereal ensures that you have a good source of protein to start the day.

Don't

There are many things you are told to avoid during pregnancy, but the biggest no-no is alcohol. It passes through the placenta to your baby and is known to have damaging effects, including affecting the baby's growth and the development of the baby's brain and central nervous system. One mother I spoke to remarked that she and her husband had always been in the habit of going out for a few drinks with colleagues after work on Fridays. When she became pregnant she stopped drinking and was amazed to find how much better she felt when she woke up on Saturday morning, and how much more she enjoyed the weekend – and this was someone who hadn't felt she drank excessively before pregnancy, so you might find yourself enjoying not drinking.

Smoking is another no-no. Mothers who smoke tend to have smaller babies that are at greater risk of complications.

The advice on the other 'don'ts' seems to change fairly frequently. They are things that effectively, in very rare circumstances, could cause upset in your digestive system and have repercussions for your baby. They are:

- **Soft cheese** such as brie and blue cheese such as gorgonzola and Roquefort, because the mould can contain listeria.

- **Raw eggs**, which carry the risk of salmonella food poisoning.

- **Pâté**, which can contain listeria.

- **Raw and undercooked meats,** taking particular care with processed meats such as sausages.

- **Raw shellfish** can cause food poisoning.

- **Tuna** (and other large fish) contain higher levels of mercury so are best avoided at all times, but particularly in pregnancy.

- **Vitamin A** in the form of retinol from meat and fish sources. (If you take vitamin A, make sure it is in the form of beta carotene from vegetable sources.)

- **Alcohol**, as it can seriously affect your baby's development.

- **Caffeine**, which is found not just in coffee but in cola and other soft drinks. Too much caffeine can cause low birth weight and, in extreme circumstances, miscarriage.

Morning sickness

If eating is an unattractive proposition in early pregnancy, it's a good idea to invest in a juicer and make juices from vegetables and fruit, so that you can more easily absorb nourishment.

Other ideas are to eat something high in protein before you go to bed at night to help keep your blood sugar levels more even, and to eat a couple of crackers or a high protein snack before you get up in the morning.

Eat small amounts of what you feel like when you feel like it. Anything (as long as it is reasonably healthy) is better than nothing, as an empty stomach can make you feel queasy.

Ginger and peppermint, taken as tea or in any other form, are both known to aid the digestion.

Take a slow, deep breath and have a rest.

The acupressure bands worn for travel sickness may help.

In my experience, supplementation with vitamin B6 capsules can work wonders.

Nutritional support

You will need a good antenatal multivitamin and mineral supplement to take during pregnancy. It is often considered wiser to take vitamins and minerals in the form of a balanced supplement rather than individually. I particularly like Prenatal from Metabolics, which is of the highest quality and has been carefully formulated to provide mothers with optimal vitamin and mineral support in a balanced formula. Prenatal is designed to provide all the nutritional support you need as described below.

It is known that folic acid, one of the B vitamins, is important in the first three months of pregnancy to help the baby's brain and spine develop. Taking folic acid reduces the risk of neural tube defects such as spina bifida.

Most of us could do with supplementation of essential fatty acids, particularly Omega 3, and this is especially important in pregnancy. Adequate levels of Omega 3 can help prevent premature labour, but it should be taken from a vegetable source such as flax seed oil.

Our hormones turn somersaults during pregnancy, and vitamin B6 can help balance the hormones and prevent morning sickness.

Magnesium is an anti-stress mineral that aids the absorption of calcium, needed for strong bones and teeth. It helps us relax, and a deficiency may contribute to post-natal depression.

It has been said that 80 per cent of the population is deficient in zinc, which is needed for growth and promotes brain and nervous system development in your baby. It is present in over 200 enzymes in the body. Zinc is a component of collagen, which is important for the connective tissue and flexibility of the body. A zinc deficiency can be a contributory factor in long labour or post-natal depression. Many of us would benefit from supplementation but particularly so when pregnant.

Your blood volume increases towards the end of pregnancy so your haemoglobin level may naturally go down because it becomes more dilute. This is perfectly normal. If you become tired as a result, it may be reaching the level where you are becoming anaemic, so your medical adviser may suggest an iron supplement. Vitamin C aids the absorption of iron, so drinking a glass of orange juice at the same time can help.

Collagen helps keep the body's connective tissue toned and flexible. Collagen supplements should not be taken during pregnancy and breastfeeding, but are an excellent way of helping your tummy get flat and firm again after you have finished breastfeeding.

Always consult a nutrition expert before taking any supplements in pregnancy.

Stretch marks

Not strictly nutrition, but stretch marks are something that concerns every pregnant woman. They are less likely to occur if you are fit, active and slim, your muscles are well toned and your diet is good. A good quality vegetable source Omega 3 supplement can aid the flexibility of your body tissue as well as the sharpness of your brain.

It is worth using a good quality stretch-mark lotion from early in pregnancy, to keep the tissue supple even before your baby's major growth spurt in the second and third trimesters. One that contains algae extract is particularly good because this encourages your body to produce collagen, to keep your stomach supple as it grows.

The importance of good nutrition

A mother's body will always tend to protect her baby, so though a developing baby will undoubtedly suffer from the effects of poor nutrition, the mother will suffer more as her body will always give her baby what it needs to the best of her ability. For instance, a woman's brain may shrink in pregnancy, not because there are fewer brain cells but because the cells may become smaller if there is a lack of essential fatty acids in the diet, and the baby takes priority for those that are available. This is just one example, but if your diet is good before and during your pregnancy, you and your baby can avoid many of the possible problems of pregnancy. Good nutrition really is important, and prevention is always better than cure.

It is important to take nutritional supplements after your baby's birth, to help you return to the nutritional status you had before you were pregnant. Many women complain of being more tired in a second pregnancy, quite possibly because they started this pregnancy at a lower nutritional status, because they had never replaced what they had lost during their first pregnancy and while breastfeeding.

Some women also complain of premenstrual tension (PMT) after their first or second pregnancies when they had never experienced it before. This too can often be rectified with appropriate nutritional support.

CHAPTER 6

Relaxation

'Nothing can bring peace but yourself.'

Ralph Waldo Emerson,
'Self-Reliance', from *Essays: First Series*, 1841

Relaxation

In this chapter I will give you some relaxations for you to practise during your pregnancy. Their main purpose is for practice before the birth. Of course you can use them as you give birth as well, but their main purpose is for practice beforehand.

Each time you practise you let go a little more and a little more of the stresses and tensions. The practice beforehand is a very important part of hypnobirthing. So many times, people have told me after their birth that if only they had realised how important it was, they would have done much more practice of the relaxations beforehand. I bite my tongue, and refrain from saying, 'But I told you so.'

D o one of these relaxations each night before you go to sleep, and just after you have done a few minutes of breathing practice. Ideally, have them read to you by your husband or partner. The only skill a father needs to be able to use these scripts extremely effectively with a mother, is to be able to read slowly and gently, and leave plenty of pauses. You may want to use some of them in early labour too, but please use them for practice beforehand, because every time you practise, you learn to relax more.

Relaxing may sound so simple, but like anything, the more we practise the better we get at it. This first script is simply a

HEAD AND FACE RELAXATION

Just allow your breathing to slow down and deepen; so comfortable and so serene. As I speak, let your eyes close gently and easily, so that you start to relax, serenely and confidently. Breathe comfortably, slowly and deeply.

Now let the relaxation in your eyelids spread outwards to your forehead so that it too relaxes and becomes smooth and comfortable. Enjoy the feeling of comfort and wellbeing.

Just pause for a short while, and now allow the relaxation to spread naturally from your forehead, flow in and around your eyes, and on downwards through your cheeks, to your jaw, and your neck – everything relaxing as the soothing comfort gently spreads.

Now allow your mouth to relax as well, so that it is entirely soft and relaxed, with your lips and your eyes gently smiling. Feel your tongue relaxing completely naturally in your mouth, so that now your whole face and head are totally and gently relaxed. Enjoy the feeling of comfort and wellbeing.

Finally, allow your shoulders to relax and sink to their natural level, so that your whole body is calm, limp and relaxed, and your breathing is soft and slow.

And now rest in the sure knowledge that this wonderful, calm relaxation is there for you when you give birth to our baby, so gently and naturally, filled with serenity and confidence.

relaxation of the head and face. We can hold a great deal of tension in our face: around our eyes, in our jaws, perhaps in our shoulders and neck. If we release the tension in the head and face, then the body relaxes in sympathy, so it helps us to release tension in the whole of the body. Relaxing the area of the jaw relates to relaxing the area of the pelvis.

So settle yourself comfortably in a quiet place, take a long, slow 'up' breath as you learnt in Chapter 3, and begin the first relaxation, the Head and Face Relaxation, on page 81.

Then open your eyes and be aware of your surroundings again. That is a lovely short relaxation.

Stroking Relaxation is another script. We live in a very untouchy society, and yet touch is so comforting and therapeutic. If you feel down, it comforts you if somebody puts their arm around your shoulders. Touch is important at any time, and it is especially important when you are giving birth. This relaxation involves your husband or partner stroking your dominant hand and arm. Start at the fingers and stroke up your hand and forearm. Stroking is relaxing on its own, but if you practise it while you are deeply relaxed, you learn to associate the touch with a much deeper relaxation than the touch on its own would carry. So when he strokes your arm while you are giving birth, it takes you into a very deep state of relaxation. This script contains five positive statements about birth. You can use all of them, or just one or two of them. Use them in a way that works for you, or use different statements on different days for variety in your daily practice.

When you practise these relaxations with your husband or partner, his voice will also become an anchor for relaxation so that, when you hear his words of encouragement, softly and gently while you are in labour, the sound of his voice will automatically take you into a state of deep relaxation.

Next we come to another script which also involves touch: Calming Touch, which begins on page 85.

At the end of each of these relaxations you can choose to either drift off to sleep or become awake and alert again. If you are using the relaxation before you go to sleep, just omit or say to yourself at the beginning that you will ignore the part that tells you to become alert, and sink into a deep and comfortable sleep.

STROKING RELAXATION

Gently and easily allow your eyes to close, so that you can focus better on my voice. Just allow your breathing to slow down and deepen ... so comfortable and so serene. Now feel the weight of your feet on the floor (or on the bed). As you focus on your feet, feel all your stress and tension flow irresistibly down out of your body through your feet, down into the ground, to be replaced by a wave of relaxation and serenity ... so you feel relief and comfort, as a feeling of warmth and wellbeing permeates your whole being. Your breath becomes slower and deeper, slower and deeper. Comfort and wellbeing.

(Start stroking her dominant hand and arm, speaking slowly and calmly.)

As I speak, I'll begin to stroke your hand very gently and softly. Just allow yourself to enjoy the pleasant sensation in your hand, the soothing, relaxing touch. Your hand feels as though it is safely enveloped in a silk or velvet glove, endorphins spreading throughout your body ... So soft, so warm, so safe, so comfortable.

Now you notice that all feeling begins to fade away from your hand. You can feel my touch, but all you are aware of in your hand is warmth and comfort, maybe a slight tingling, and your hand becomes increasingly numb. It rests relaxed, loose and senseless ... As I keep stroking, so the feeling in your hand becomes less and less, and you feel so relaxed, because you know your hand is completely safe and comfortable. Gradually your hand becomes completely free from sensation ... until you feel nothing at all in your hand.

Now you can apply this warm, comfortable numbness

Continued overleaf...

... *Continued from page 83*

wherever you wish to in your body. All you have to do is just bring to mind the part of your body that will be free from sensation, and all feeling gradually fades gently away, fades gently away. Enjoy this sensation. Comfort and wellbeing. As you are now very relaxed, just spend a little time to:

1 Allow a feeling of wellbeing and empowerment to permeate your body, and fill you with confidence at the birth of your baby.
2 Appreciate the power of your maternal intuition, that guides and protects you and your baby through labour and birth.
3 Grow in confidence knowing that your body has been made to give birth efficiently and calmly.
4 Allow your body to loosen and relax, as you do during your labour and your baby's natural birth.
5 Allow your mind and body to grow in harmony for a swift and gentle labour and birth.

(Pause. When enough time has passed, stop stroking, and bring her back to normality, talking in a normal voice at a normal volume.)

This has been a very special time as you are so relaxed and happy in the knowledge of the fulfilment that is before you, in the birth of our baby. You now know you are able to affect your body as you wish. In a minute it will be time to come back to me in this room, bringing the calm confidence with you, wonderfully relaxed, refreshed and empowered, confident that our baby's birth will be relaxed and healthy, calm and quick. Knowing that, next time we do this, you will relax even more deeply, your confidence will be even more profound, and you will quickly become even more free of all sensation ... And now, in your own time, open your eyes – wide awake and alert.

CALMING TOUCH

(Gently rest your hand on the wrist of your wife or partner's dominant hand.)

As my hand rests on your wrist, so your eyes close, and your eyelids rest just as lightly, just as gently on your cheeks. You feel relief as the area around your eyes relaxes, more and more deeply, and that feeling of comfort and relaxation spreads out across your forehead, around your temples, flowing gently down, passing your cheekbones, and your jaws, so soft, so easy. Now feel the relaxation growing, and including your neck and your shoulders, and your whole body sinks into deep and comfortable relaxation, deeper and deeper, so comfortable, so easy; a wonderful feeling of wellbeing.

Now observe that your breathing has slowed … and deepened. Breathing in … and breathing out, breathing in … and breathing out … Deeper and deeper … so comfortable, so serene.

Now I shall easily raise your arm a little *(raise her arm about 15 to 30cm)*. Notice how heavy and limp it feels. It feels very, very good just to allow me to lift your arm, knowing that, in a minute, when I gently allow it to drop, your relaxation will deepen more and more *(release her arm)*.

Now again, just notice your arm rising easily as I raise it *(raise arm)*. And when I drop it your relaxation will be very, very deep *(release arm)*. So deeply relaxed. Deeper and deeper.

And again, now, I'm gently raising your arm *(raise arm)*. As I let go, you go many times deeper *(release arm)*. Deeper and deeper. More and more relaxed. So comfortable. So profound.

Continued overleaf…

... *Continued from page 85*

Enjoy this unique comfort and depth of relaxation that you have created in your body and mind. Deeper and deeper. Know now that this easy, deep relaxation is there for you as you, your body, and your baby share the empowering experience of labour and birth, gently, confidently, calmly.

Allow this feeling of intuitive calm to remain with you as I count from five to one and you gradually become aware of your surroundings again.

Five ... notice the energy begin to flow gently in. Four ... the beginnings of alertness. Three ... now some gentle movements start again. Two ... noticing the sounds around you, and one ... eyes open, calm, aware, awake and confident, both now and when you calmly and gently give birth to your baby.

You can read the following script, Colour and Calmness, for yourself, or have it read to you last thing at night. It's also available on a CD, as are all the other relaxations in this book; see the back of this book for details. Colour and Calmness is simply a lovely relaxation to use as you drift off to sleep each night.

COLOUR AND CALMNESS

It's so simple to let your breathing be completely natural, and notice just how easily and gently you are relaxing, breathing in and breathing out ... breathing in and breathing out ... deeply, slowly, comfortably.

As you relax more deeply, you notice that your eyelids feel heavier, and very naturally start closing ... slowly and easily ... slowly and easily ... until now they are completely closed.

Now give yourself permission to imagine a warm, unstoppable wave of complete relaxation, starting at the very top of your head, and beginning to wash comfortably down through your body. As it flows through every part of your body, so that part becomes completely limp and relaxed. Feel it now flowing from the top of your head down. Your forehead becomes completely smooth as it totally relaxes.

Now you feel the muscles around your eyes soften and release. Now your cheeks relax ... now your lips ... and even inside your mouth, your tongue relaxes. Now the muscles of your jaw soften and let go ... comfortably ... easily ... as you go down and further down ... enjoy the release.

The wave flows on through your neck, relaxing it and enveloping your shoulders, and now that feeling of warmth and ease washes down your arms, relaxing every point as it flows from your shoulders, through your upper arms, past your elbows, down into your lower arms, and on into your hands, the back of your hands and your palms, all the way down to the ends of your fingers, allowing everything to become relaxed and comfortable.

Now the wave surges gently on through your chest,

Continued overleaf...

... *Continued from page 87*

relaxing everything, through your stomach, gently soothing ... and you feel the muscles of your pelvic area relax, just as they will as you give birth to your baby ... and on into your legs, down your thighs, and into your lower legs, then down into your feet, where, like the surging sea, it laps at the very tips of your toes, making both your legs completely relaxed. And now you realise that you are very, very relaxed. This feeling of wellbeing allows you to go deeper, down and further down, and each time you go more quickly, more deeply, easily and gently into ultimate relaxation. Down and further down. More and more profound.

Now you become even more deeply relaxed, as you imagine yourself in a warm and crystal clear sea, and you find that you can breathe just as easily underwater as on the surface, and so you let yourself gently and safely sink down and further down into the warm, comfortable water, observing all the beautiful coral and fish of every colour and hue, shape and size. And as you sink deeper, you become more and more profoundly relaxed, until you find yourself on the bottom, lying gently on the soft sand, surrounded by all these beautiful colours, and completely, completely, relaxed and calm.

As you lie comfortably, calmly and relaxed on the warm, soft sand, breathing easily, deeply, slowly, happily and calmly, you notice that, as the different shoals of fish come and go, twist and turn, change shape and intermingle, they create the most beautiful patterns and colours, and these colours affect your own emotions with their beauty, and your body and mind absorb their calmness and fluidity, allowing you to sink down and further down, into gentle peace.

And now you notice that, almost miraculously, the different-coloured fish have separated into bands of colour, so that, like light through a prism, every colour of the spectrum can be seen before you, gently pulsating to the rhythm of your body, as the fish themselves gently twist and turn. How relaxing this is; so calming and so peaceful.

Now the fish swirl silently, separate and move away out of sight, until, like a soft cloud, you see coming towards you the most beautiful purple shoal of gentle, dainty fish, ranging in colour from a soft red to a calming blue. And as the fish surround you and pass around each other, you experience the energy of the colour purple, flowing softly around and through you, bringing you confidence and trust. This has a wonderful effect on your mind, filling you with relaxation, and happiness, and serenity, bringing you the peace of mind that will be with you throughout your pregnancy, and your baby's birth. So you feel calm and confident, and these wonderful feelings allow you to trust your inner wisdom, and drift down and further down, safer and safer.

See before you now the red fish separating and leaving as a body, off into the distance, and almost miraculously the colour surrounding and permeating you becomes the wonderful blue of the shoal that remains, clear and serene like the azure blueness of a summer's day, and this blue flows softly around and through the upper part of your body, bringing a lightness and beauty to your world, and with it a gentle and soft happiness. A feeling of calmness, peace and wellbeing envelopes and soothes you, down and further down.

You notice that your breathing becomes even more gentle and easy, and this wonderful blue is in complete harmony with the area of your neck, your shoulders, and your throat, as they relax more and more, and become softer and softer. You use gentle and positive words, in your inner conversations and when you

Continued overleaf...

... *Continued from page 89*

speak to your baby, and you feel as though all your muscles have completely softened. You feel relaxed and weightless ... a profound feeling of wellbeing and trust.

Now a group of yellow fish silently joins the blue fish, which turns the colour around you to the gentle green of spring, the time of new beginnings, just as your body is so naturally and healthily vibrant with new life, and this mingling of the yellow and blue fish, each vanishing as separate colours, permeates you with the energy of green, a green that gladdens and relaxes your heart itself, where you feel such joy and love now, and deepens even further your calmness and relaxation. Joy and love for your baby envelop you, and you experience a deeper connection with this new, small being. With the new, gentle green you feel so close to Nature as she caresses and enfolds you. You are wholly enveloped with that wonderful feeling of calmness and relaxation which Nature brings to all she touches – down and further down.

Notice now that the blue fish are drifting away, all together, and only the yellow fish remain, like a shimmering meadow of yellow flowers, which brings peace and calm throughout the centre of your body. You feel the fish swimming gently around you, never touching, but the faint tremor of the water as they move caresses the centre of your body, and seems to flow right through you, drawing you into a state of yet deeper relaxation and harmony, down and further down, as your breathing becomes even more effortless and gentle, your muscles loose, and your body at ease.

And then you notice that the shoal is turning almost imperceptibly but smoothly into a soft orange, like the flesh of a melon, as a new shoal of red fish arrives and intermingles with the yellow ones, changing the colour from yellow to orange as their numbers increase. You feel this colour change particularly affects your abdomen, which softens even further, and relaxes, as every element within it calms and softens, and you become even more closely connected to the baby you feel growing within you. This effect soothes and softens your body throughout the area of your abdomen, and so you become more and more relaxed ready for the birth of your baby, as your mind and body move closer and closer together in serenity and peace. Down and further down.

But now the colours of the fish change yet again as the shoal of yellow fish swims away, so that all becomes a deep, soft red, bringing great calmness and relaxation which permeates your pelvic area and the lower part of your body. You are full of confidence and trust. You are calm, and peaceful, and happy, and you feel that the future holds good things for you, so you trust in nature, trust in your intuition, and trust in the natural process of pregnancy, labour and birth. You know that your body is designed to give birth naturally, and work with your baby during its smooth passage into the world. These wonderful feelings allow you to drift down and further down, safer and safer, encompassing your entire body, mind and spirit.

Now something wonderful happens. The red fish in their shimmering haze quietly move away from you out of sight, and you notice that the dappled light, filtering through the ripples of the water, has changed the sand you are lying on to a soft bed of purest white, as if all the colours that have passed around you have left behind their very essence, and produced their natural combination of white light, on which you now

Continued overleaf...

... *Continued from page 91*

rest, so gently that you can hardly feel it at all, so gently
that you feel the softness saturating your very being. This
feeling of peacefulness, relaxation, and confident and
instinctive happiness, reminds you that the happiness
and joy of a natural, swift, healthy and calm birth, for
you and for your baby, is just as natural as all the colours
of the beautiful, gentle fish that have swirled around you
and enveloped you with their fluid softness, and is equally
a part of nature.

So now you know that all is well; all is very well. You
know that your labour and birth are a completely natural
process in the way that nature intended ... and you carry
within you the memory of this wonderful experience of the
colours and calmness.

This has been very pleasant, so it is completely natural for
you to pass from this experience to a deep and happy sleep,
waking at the right time, joyful, refreshed, and relaxed, and
looking forward with confidence and trust to your baby
arriving so naturally, gently and calmly. If that is how you
would like this session to end, just slip off to sleep now.

If you would like to come back to a state of alertness,
then follow my instructions, and the energy will easily and
naturally flow back into you. I will start counting now. Five
... starting to become aware of my count. Four ... slowly
taking control of your muscles again. Three ... feel the
energy begin to flow back into your body. Two ... noticing
the sounds around you, and one ... finally your eyes gently
open, and you feel happy, refreshed and very calm.

Filled with confidence and trust in your body and in the
natural process of birth.

Positive birth statements

Overleaf are some statements to empower you ready to give birth to your baby with confidence. These positive statements about birth are very simple and remarkably effective. You can listen to them or read them yourself, either silently or aloud. Use the different senses in your practice: visual if you are reading them for yourself; auditory if your husband or partner is reading them aloud to you, or if you are reading them aloud to yourself, or if you are listening to them on a CD or on your iPhone.

You don't have to read all the statements at once; you can just read a few of them one time, and then a few more another time. If there is one statement that you particularly like, write it out and put it on a piece of paper in your pocket or your handbag, and then you can bring it out and read it during the day.

One couple I taught had a blackboard for the shopping list in their kitchen, and sometimes the father would come down first in the morning and write one of the positive statements on the blackboard ready for when his wife came down. A few days later he would change the words as a surprise for her.

You could also write some of them in colourful letters on large sheets of paper, and put them up on a wall so you will see them as you go past. You could put different statements around the house and change them from time to time. It's all good practice and it all works well.

STATEMENTS FOR AN EMPOWERING BIRTH

- **I move gently** forward through my pregnancy and labour with confidence and trust.

- **I see my baby's birth** as natural, healthy, swift and easy.

- **I am practising** so that I am relaxed and calm during labour.

- **Birthing is a natural process** of my body, my mind and my spirit, working in unison with my baby.

- **I acknowledge and trust** the innate wisdom of my body and my intuition to guide me through pregnancy, labour and the birth of my baby.

- **I trust the instinctive** process of birth, which flows naturally through my body.

- **My mind leads** where my body follows. As my mind is so relaxed, confident and calm, so my body is comfortable, relaxed, soft and open, as my baby passes gently, healthily and swiftly into the world.

- **As I feel my baby** moving inside me, my love and connection grow ever deeper.

- **I approach my baby's birth** with optimism and confidence.

- **I practise profound relaxation,** and I deepen my confidence and trust.

- **I am secure in the knowledge** that I am fully prepared for a natural, easy and swift birth.

- **I have confidence** that a natural birth is safe for me, and safe for my baby.

- **I choose the best possible** caregivers during my pregnancy and the birth of my baby.

- **I choose the best place** for my baby to be born naturally and calmly.

- **I enjoy the feeling** of natural calm, relaxation and softness that permeates my body.

- **As I gently progress** through labour and birth, I go deeper into relaxation and calmness.

- **Each breath is slow,** long, deep and relaxed.

- **With each surge** I breathe deeply, focus upwards, and work with my body.

- **With each breath out,** I breathe out tension and stress.

- **With each breath in,** I breathe in relaxation and comfort, peace and trust.

- **I feel positive,** confident and optimistic, and I look forward to my baby's birth.

- **Throughout my labour** I go deeper and deeper within to my innate wisdom and intuition.

- **I flow with the natural rhythms** of my body, which gently and swiftly ease my baby into the world.

- **I trust that my body** and my baby are healthy, relaxed and calm.

- **My baby naturally moves** into the best position for a natural, swift and gentle birth.

- **I eat healthily** and take care of my body for me and for my baby.

- **My body and my baby's body** are created the right size to birth naturally.

- **My baby is born** at the right time for a natural, swift and gentle birth.

... Continued from page 95

■ **I trust the natural process** of birth working gently through my body and my baby.

■ **Each surge of my body** reminds me that I will soon be holding my baby in my arms.

■ **I serenely accept my birthing** as just right for me, and for my baby.

■ **I relax more and more deeply** as my labour advances and my baby moves closer and closer to birth.

■ **I feel calm,** relaxed and at ease.

■ **With each surge** my breath is slow and deep, my body is relaxed, and my mind is calm.

■ **I trust my body,** my instinct, and nature to lead me and my baby gently through labour and birth.

■ **As labour develops,** my relaxation deepens and my body softens and opens, wider and wider.

■ **After my baby is born,** gently, calmly and healthily, the placenta follows easily and naturally.

■ **My baby moves smoothly** into the world, the placenta follows, and my blood vessels close naturally and healthily.

■ **I have plenty of milk** for my baby, and I feed my baby easily and comfortably.

■ **My baby feeds well** from me and thrives.

■ **My body is designed** to give birth efficiently and easily.

■ **I have chosen to be relaxed,** calm and confident during labour.

■ **My baby is born** healthy, alert and serene.

■ **I welcome my baby** with love and delight.

CHAPTER 7

Responsibility and Choices

❧

'A little child enters your life and fills a place in your heart. A place you never knew was empty.'

Anon.

Responsibility and Choices

The birth recommendations from the World Health Organization (WHO) are worth discussing. The recommendations are known as the 'Fortelesa Declaration' and come from a report on Appropriate Technology for Birth, published by the WHO in 1985. The report starts with the phrase 'Birth is not an illness', which we would do well to remember.

The recommendations are based on the principle that each woman has a fundamental right to receive proper antenatal care; that she has a central role in all aspects of this care including participation in the planning, carrying out and evaluation of the care; and that social, emotional and psychological factors are decisive in the understanding and implementation of proper antenatal care. This seems to be a simple, obvious and fundamental principle regarding women's rights during pregnancy and birth, but very often a mother doesn't actually receive this proper care. We talk quite a lot in this book about the alternatives available to you, simply because you may not be told them otherwise. This is not necessarily to say that the alternatives are better, but simply so that you are informed. You need to know what your choices are, and be able to discuss them sensibly with your medical advisers, so that you can make the decisions that are best for you. Here are the WHO's recommendations.

1 The whole community should be informed about various procedures in birth care, to enable each woman to choose the type of birth care she prefers.
So often a woman will say to me, 'Nobody told me about a homebirth', 'I'm not allowed to do this', or 'They say I've got to do that.' Where has the choice gone?

2 The training of professional midwives or birth attendants should be promoted. Care during normal pregnancy and birth and following birth should be the duty of this profession.
As you probably know, in the United States there are some states where midwives are illegal. The birth attendant has to be an obstetrician. Both professions have their place of course, but midwives are the experts in *natural* birth. In the UK we are extremely lucky that most births are conducted by midwives.

3 Information about birth practices in hospitals (rates of Caesarean section, etc.) should be given to the public to be served by the hospital.
In the UK you can kind find this information at www.birthchoiceuk.com.

4 There is no justification in any specific geographic region to have more than a 10 to 15 per cent rate of births by Caesarean section.
In the UK the Caesarean rate is approaching 30 per cent; in some parts of the United States it is moving towards 40 per cent. I understand that in Colombia it is 95 per cent in private hospitals. In Japan and South Africa it is very high. At The Farm, which is Ina May Gaskin's natural birth centre in Tennessee, it is 1.4 per cent. Caesarean sections are wonderful in emergencies; they save lives. But when you consider the

miracle that is our bodies, how can it be that 30 per cent of women have bodies which cannot perform a function they are designed to perform? That is, to give birth.

5 There is no evidence that a Caesarean section is required after a previous transverse lower segment Caesarean section birth. Vaginal deliveries after Caesarean sections should normally be encouraged wherever emergency service or capacity is available.
This is a very interesting statement because the assumption is so often that one Caesarean section leads to another – although this view is gradually changing.

6 There is no evidence that routine foetal monitoring during labour has a positive effect on the outcome of pregnancy.
I wonder how many women in labour have been told to lie flat on their backs in the least comfortable position, with the threat that they are putting their baby's life at risk if they do not agree to having a monitor strapped to their abdomen, with a machine bleeping the heart rate beside them. All these things have their place. It is the word 'routine' that is the problem.

7 There is no evidence that pubic shaving or pre-delivery enema is advantageous.
This doesn't happen in the UK anymore, but it does happen in many other countries.

8 Pregnant women should not be put in the lithotomy position during labour or delivery. They should be encouraged to walk during labour and each woman must decide freely which position to adopt during delivery.

The lithotomy position is flat on your back with your legs in stirrups – the 'stranded beetle' position. Again, fortunately, this practice is not used routinely in the UK, though possibly it still does happen more often than it should. In some countries it is still standard practice. I see no reason why a woman should particularly be encouraged to walk. It could waste energy that she would do better to conserve for giving birth to her baby. She can do whatever she feels like.

9 The systematic use of episiotomy is not justified.
Episiotomy is when the perineum is surgically cut to make a larger opening for the baby to pass through. It is not systematically used in the UK, though of course there are times when it saves lives. There are some countries where the practice is still absolutely standard. How can it be thought that a woman needs to be cut to get her baby out when her body was designed to do it perfectly well?

10 Birth should not be induced for convenience, and the induction of labour should be reserved for specific medical indications. No geographic region should have rates of induction over 10 per cent.
In the UK the rate is about 20 per cent and we will talk about induction later on.

11 The routine administration of analgesic or anaesthetic drugs that are not specifically required to correct or prevent a complication in delivery should be avoided.
This recommendation makes sense, but there are some countries where it is standard practice to give drugs, although of course, it is wonderful that pain-relieving drugs are available if they are needed. The question is why should they be needed? Birth is a natural event, which is what hypnobirthing is all about.

12 Artificial early rupture of the membrane as a routine process is not scientifically justified.

Breaking the waters artificially is not done *routinely* in the UK, although it is still very common in UK delivery suites where, due to pressure on resources, medical staff may have to process women through the system quickly. The birth rate in the UK has risen considerably in the last ten years, but resources and the number of midwives haven't. Artificial rupture of the membrane is rarely used at home or in midwife-led units (birth centres) because it can cause complications. Again, it is the word 'routine' that is the problem.

13 The healthy newborn must remain with the mother wherever both of their conditions permit it. No process of observation of the healthy newborn justifies a separation from the mother.

This recommendation is becoming increasingly well known. That first hour of life is very precious; it is the time when the mother and baby bond, and they should never be disturbed unless there is a medical emergency. Some hospitals are even starting to encourage proper skin-to-skin contact of mother and baby in the operating theatre after a Caesarean delivery, although lots of warm blankets over both are needed as operating theatres are kept cool to reduce the risk of infection.

14 The immediate beginning of breastfeeding should be promoted even before the mother leaves the delivery room.

Every other mammal feeds as soon as it is born: lambs do, calves do, and human babies are programmed to as well. It is the time when breastfeeding starts most easily and naturally. Babies have been observed to suck in utero; mothers produce milk. Put the two together and you get breastfeeding. It's as simple and natural as that. A baby that is immediately put on its mother's chest at birth will tend to do a 'chest crawl' and find the nipple itself within about the first 20 minutes after birth, and start to feed all on its own. It is thought that the baby is probably guided by a sense of smell in performing this entirely natural action.

15 Obstetric care services that have critical attitudes towards technology and that have adopted an attitude of respect for the emotional, psychological and social aspects of birth should be identified. Such services should be encouraged and the processes that have led them to their position must be studied so that they can be used as models to foster similar attitudes in other centres and to influence obstetrical views nationwide.

This principle is so obvious, and absolutely true. Sometimes care services promote natural birth; sometimes they don't. In general, progress is encouraging, and the trend towards natural birth is gathering pace, though there is still a long way to go.

16 Governments should consider developing regulations to permit the use of new birth technologies only after adequate evaluation.

Sometimes, when you look at the research that has or hasn't been done, and the procedures that take place absolutely routinely, you just wish that this kind of evaluation would happen soon. Ultrasound scanning, the continuous monitoring of the foetal heart during labour, and the administration of vitamin K to the baby after birth are procedures that have been introduced without adequate research on the assumption they would only do good, and they have even become routine.

Who is responsible for my baby's birth?

All this is food for a great deal of thought, and leads us to the question, 'Who is responsible for your baby's birth?' And the answer is – you. Mothers who come to hypnobirthing for a gentle birth, come because it works well; but it is a partnership, between you, your husband or partner, and your medical advisers. Of course, you treat the knowledge and experience of your medical advisors with the greatest respect, but ultimately your body and your baby are your responsibility.

In a big, busy modern hospital there will be something like 6,000 births a year. A week after your baby is born, it is unlikely that anyone will remember you; but you will remember the experience for the whole of the rest of your life – and so will your baby. Therefore, it is only you who has an exclusive vested interest in the birth being as you would like it to be. People in the midwifery and obstetric professions want to support you, but they do have other pressures as well. You may be fortunate in all the circumstances of your baby's birth, but if you are clear about how you can achieve the best possible birth, and remain focused on this aim, then the mind leads and the body follows. It is amazing how often what you focus on becomes a reality.

It is worth remembering that birth is a natural process, and if you create the most natural environment, you are setting the stage for it to progress easily. As a mother your instincts are powerful and right. Follow your intuition about where and how you want your baby's birth to be. Your job is to focus on the birth you want.

Sometimes mothers get diverted by the 'what-ifs' and 'just in cases'. 'What if that happens?' 'I'm going to do this just in case.' But you have a midwife to consider the what-ifs and just-in-cases: that is part of her job. If you focus on what might go wrong, that's where your mind will tend to lead you. Focus on what you want and let the midwife deal with the what-ifs. She is trained in what-ifs. Most of the 'what-ifs' are very rare. I am not suggesting you bury your head in the sand and pretend they don't exist. Inform yourself, consider them, make your decision, and then set them aside and focus on the positive and on where you want to be.

A woman in labour goes into herself and she is not in a place to negotiate with anyone. She enters what midwives call her 'birth trance' – an altered state of consciousness created and supported by being undisturbed, quiet and observed as little as possible, so her birth hormones flow freely and well. It has been said that the best environment for a baby's conception is also the best environment for a baby's birth. Her husband or partner who also understands the principle of calm and natural birth and is prepared to speak for her clearly, calmly and courageously, can make all the difference between an unhappy and an empowering experience. The person who is with you during labour is extremely important. To have the right caregiver is beyond price.

The father's role

Fathers used not to be allowed at the birth of their child, which now seems almost unbelievable. These days a father is almost expected to be there, which can also cause problems. Many fathers want to be at the birth, and some do not. Many mothers want to have their husband or partner supporting them at the birth, and some would prefer to have their mother or sister there. It is important to do what's right for you. There is a theory that a father is an unhelpful influence in the birthing room, but that does not apply to hypnobirthing fathers. Many women say, 'I couldn't have done it without him.'

If the father is frightened, doesn't know what's going on, doesn't know what to do to help, feels rather responsible, and is producing fear hormones, he is negatively affecting the environment. On the other hand, a father who has learnt hypnobirthing with his wife, has practised with her, and is producing the hormones of confidence and calm, is positively affecting the environment. Being a supportive part of the process of his baby being born can enrich and deepen the couple's relationship and also deepen the relationship between him and his child, because he knows that he played an important part in the birth process, which is the most formative experience of our lives.

It's also true that people talk a lot, and quite rightly, about a mother during pregnancy and how her hormones change. But the father's hormones change, too. Dr Sarah J. Buckley, author of *Gentle Birth, Gentle Mothering,* tells us that a father's level of the hormone prolactin rises just before the birth, leading to prolactin being called 'the hormone of paternity', and fathers with a higher level of prolactin are more responsive to the cries of a newborn. One new study has suggested that men's testosterone levels drop steeply after becoming a father. A mother's instinct is to nurture, and a father's instinct is to protect. These roles are not exclusive, but the instinct to protect becomes much heightened in the father during late pregnancy.

I see this sometimes in the questions that come up in a hypnobirthing class. A mother will tell me in the break that she would really like to have her baby at home but her partner doesn't want her to. Her instinct to nurture is guiding her to a small, safe place to give birth, and home is her safe place. His instinct to protect is telling him that it's his responsibility to make sure she and the baby are safe, and he is programmed from an early age to think that giving birth in hospital is safer. It looks as if they're in disagreement, but that is not really the case. They both want the same thing: the best possible birth for their child.

I once asked a group of fathers what it was that they feared about homebirth. Was it the mess? There is surprisingly little mess, and the midwife clears it up, so that wasn't the real problem. Was it that the baby might arrive before the midwife? That was a slight concern but it wasn't really a major problem because it seldom happens. Was the problem the birthing pool – the floor might collapse under its weight? It has been pointed out that if ten people could be in your room having a party then the floor certainly won't collapse because of a birthing pool, and two women in stiletto heels standing on one floor joist could be putting greater pressure on that joist than the diffused weight of a pool over the whole floor. It transpired in the end that the real problem was fear of the unknown. The fathers didn't quite know what to expect. It is a common fear, similar to when someone is afraid of the dark: it's not the dark they're afraid of, but what might be in it that they can't quite see – the unknown.

If a couple appear to have a difference of opinion, it is probably due to lack of information. Do some research. Find out what the facts are, and you will probably find that you both come to the same conclusion. In hypnobirthing a father is hugely important and can make a great difference to the birth, deepening the couple's relationship and his relationship with his child.

Midwives and obstetricians

Both midwives and obstetricians are autonomous professionals. Before I started to teach hypnobirthing, I had the idea that midwives were dear, sweet things, who had a basic medical knowledge and were very supportive of mothers and babies. In fact, midwives do a three-year degree course. Their medical knowledge is superb. They care for mothers antenatally, while they give birth, and after the baby is born. They are highly trained in natural birth and know how to facilitate it, how to bring it back on course if something is slightly out of the ordinary, and when to call in an obstetrician if extra help is needed. Midwives, in my experience, are almost always extremely supportive of hypnobirthing because their whole ethos is to support a mother giving birth, and they have seen the difference that hypnobirthing makes. The reports I get from mothers are almost always that 'the midwife was wonderful'. So all the 'what-ifs' or 'just-in-cases' that may be on your mind can be safely left to a midwife: they are highly qualified, very knowledgeable, and have had an intensive, technical training.

Obstetricians, on the other hand, are taught to deal with the emergencies. When they are training they are called in to observe and help with any complicated births, as well as simply to attend some normal births. They do not usually care for a woman through her labour, unless there are unusual circumstances, but are called in right at the end. They will do Caesarean sections, forceps deliveries, ventouse (vacuum extraction) deliveries, and they will be called in when something out of the ordinary happens. Therefore, obstetricians have a different view of birth from midwives and parents.

I remember being phoned one day by a mother who was also a doctor and who was planning to do a hypnobirthing class. She said, 'I know I have a skewed view of birth because I've only ever seen emergencies, but I'm scared.' Almost all doctors will never have seen a homebirth, so a doctor or an obstetrician's view will tend to be that birth is a medical emergency, because that is their reality and experience.

A midwife views birth much more as a normal, natural event where occasionally some extra help is needed. In her training a midwife must support mothers in at least 40 normal births as well as assisting in another 40 less-than-straightforward births, among many other tasks. We are lucky in the UK to have midwives supporting mothers as they give birth. We are also lucky to have good obstetricians available when they are needed. Both are autonomous professionals who have their own role to play. A midwife is not an obstetric nurse who is an assistant to the obstetrician; she has her own professional role.

Be sure that your medical advisers will be unwaveringly supportive of how you want your birth to be. If you are giving birth in a hospital or midwife-led unit, it may be possible to ask for a different midwife if the chemistry is just not right between you. If a stressful situation arises during the antenatal stage, an appointment with the senior midwife to talk it through can be helpful. Be prepared to change to another midwife if necessary to make sure you feel comfortable.

Independent midwives

Employing an independent midwife ensures that you are cared for by an experienced midwife whom you will know well. Independent midwives are fully qualified and registered with the Nursing and Midwifery Council, the same as an NHS midwife. Her visits will last as long as you need, all your questions will be answered, and she will continue to visit you after your baby is born. Mothers have described it as 'a priceless service' and 'the best money I ever spent', so it is worth calling one or two independent midwives who live near you to find out some more. Have a look on the website www.independentmidwives.org.uk.

Doulas

Some women will employ a doula to be with them during the birth of their baby. The word 'doula' comes from the

Greek word meaning female slave. A doula is not medically qualified but she is trained to support the mother, giving her confidence, being her advocate, perhaps giving the father time to rest, and generally she will have a greater knowledge of the birth process, hospital procedures, and what will make the mother comfortable. It is a role that midwives would love to perform but these days they are highly qualified medical professionals who are often too busy to be able to just be with the mothers in their care. Hypnobirthing fathers are well equipped to be supportive themselves, but some couples feel that having a doula gives them extra reassurance.

Taking a central role

Taking responsibility for your baby's birth includes everything that makes up your internal and external environment in body, mind and spirit. Make sure you have only positive and helpful people around you.

Being a parent is a position of great importance and responsibility. You are entitled to be treated with the greatest respect in this role. The choices that you make now will have an effect on the development and serenity of your baby. Choose wisely.

CHAPTER 8

Achieving the Birth You Want

'The parallels between making love and giving birth are clear, not only in terms of passion and love, but also because we need essentially the same conditions for both experiences: privacy and safety.'

Dr Sarah J. Buckley,
Gentle Birth, Gentle Mothering, 2009

Achieving the Birth You Want

When I started to teach hypnobirthing, I received many wonderful stories from mothers whose babies were born calmly and naturally, but sometimes I was told about births that were not what a mother had hoped for. When this happened I considered very carefully if I could learn something that would help other mothers in future. I came to realise that very often in these births there had been some form of medical intervention.

Couples need information on all the alternatives in order to make an informed decision. The law in the UK says that no intervention may be done without informed consent. So often, however, the only information given is about why the routine procedures should be agreed to, and the consent can be assumed.

I am well aware that the wonders of modern medicine save lives. The problem is that some interventions are done routinely when a mother would do better to remember that, very often, baby knows best.

The due date

Let's talk now about due dates. They can be a snare and a delusion, and the cause of extreme stress. In the early 1800s a German obstetrician, Franz Naegele, declared that a pregnancy should last for ten moons (ten months of four weeks). However, researchers in 1990 found that, for healthy Eurasian women, an average pregnancy is ten days longer than this. So the due date is not even an average.

Nothing in the human condition is standard. We all grow to different heights, live different length lives, we have different faces, different coloured hair; it would be strange indeed if all pregnancies were the same length. Even if you look at the apples on an apple tree, they take over a month to ripen, and if you want one to ripen early and pick the ripest and put it on a sunny windowsill in the kitchen, guess what? The ones on the tree ripen first.

The more I see of birth, the more I am in absolute awe of how everything has been thought of, and I am firmly of the opinion that you disturb it at your peril. Of course there are circumstances when we are extremely grateful for medical intervention. In particular medical circumstances, intervention saves lives. But there seems to be a tremendous amount of it these days, and we should regard it with great caution.

In the UK, a full-term pregnancy is generally considered to be 40 weeks. In France, it is considered to be 41 weeks. In Kenya, it is up to 43 weeks. The World Health Organization says anything between 37 and 42 weeks, which is more than a month's range for a normal pregnancy. The length of pregnancy will vary because the length of pregnancy is taken from the first day of the woman's last menstrual period. A woman may have an irregular menstrual cycle, or she might not know exactly when she conceived because women can conceive at different times. There are so many factors to take into account. Scans, too, are not 100 per cent accurate. The date given by an ultrasound scan in the first trimester of pregnancy tells us how long the baby has been growing for, plus or minus five days. Most women have an anomaly scan at 20 weeks, which is accurate to plus or minus ten days. Maybe it would be healthier to take the view that there is no such thing as a 'late baby', but that some women simply have a natural length of pregnancy of 42 weeks or sometimes even more.

When the arbitrary 'due date' comes along and your baby hasn't arrived (and most won't have arrived by then), the stress begins to build. You will find that it comes from three sides.

You put stress on yourself, because you have mentally set great store on that date. This is why I would suggest that, if your baby is due, say, on 1 May, every time that date comes into your mind you say to yourself, 'My baby is due in the first half of May'. Reading this book now, it may be difficult to imagine how stressed you will feel, but it is very likely you will, so it is wise to protect yourself from it. Some midwives have suggested that, rather than having a 'due date', you have a best-before date at 42 weeks, which takes a lot of the pressure off you.

You will have stress from your family and friends. When that date comes you will get 20 phone calls. 'Baby hasn't come yet?' 'No.' 'You're still there?' 'Yes' – of course you are or you wouldn't be answering the phone. 'You must be fed up' – 'I wasn't until you suggested it to me.' Many mothers have unplugged the phone to stem the mounting tide of phone calls. To protect yourself from these well-meaning but stress-provoking enquiries, you can tell each of your friends a different date. They don't really mind when your baby will arrive; it's simply polite to ask. Tell the first friend 14 May, and the second 13 May, etc. When they ask you again next week and you tell them a different date, they probably won't remember what you told them last week. If they do, you can simply say that you had another scan and they changed the date. Or else tell everyone a date at 42 weeks to protect yourself.

Here is some advice from a father:

> Based on our experience, patience is paramount. Different strategies may be used to avoid unnecessary pressure. The best one I can think of is keeping the due date a secret. When asked, give the end of the 42nd week as the due date. Everyone, family and friends, wants to have a date and no matter how many times you tell them not to keep asking about whether the baby has arrived or not, chances are at least one of them will not get the message and that will be enough. Being vague is pointless and will not satisfy everyone. It's much easier to publicise the 'wrong' date.

Third and last, you will have stress from the medical profession. What often happens at your first antenatal visit following this fictitious due date, is that the hospital will say, 'We induce at term plus ten days. We don't allow you to go beyond ten days.' If there is a particular medical indication, then an induction is justified, but the word 'allow' is not. It is a mother's decision whether to be induced. In any other sphere of medicine, a line of treatment is proposed, discussed and it is up to the patient to decide whether they want to go down that path. Yet it seems that often a pregnant woman is not treated with this degree of respect.

The reason for this policy is that there is a higher stillbirth rate at 43 weeks than at 40 weeks, but there is no research which shows that the cause of this increase is the longer pregnancy. But the research is invariably interpreted this way, and a pregnant woman will often be asked, 'Don't you want to do the best for your baby?' Pressure like that simply puts a mother under stress. When she is under stress she is in the fear response. She cannot be in the fear response and the confident response at the same time. In the confident response, as we saw in Chapter 2, she is producing oxytocin and is more likely to go into labour. The more pressure she is put under, the less likely she is to go into labour.

The other reason for this policy is the theory that the placenta can fail. Please note, the placenta can fail, not the placenta *will* fail. If a placenta starts to fail it gradually becomes less efficient, so it makes sense to be monitored daily or every other day, if you prefer not to be induced at the standard time specified by your hospital. Mothers are also often told that their baby will grow too big to be born normally if it stays in the womb 'too long'. This is a little hard to square with the previous statement that the placenta may fail. How can a baby grow 'too big' if the placenta is becoming less efficient in giving it nourishment?

If a baby is born outside the 37–42 week period, the baby may still be perfectly normal and healthy. It is a perfectly viable option to monitor the mother and baby beyond 42 weeks to make sure both are healthy and well and the pregnancy is progressing normally. If all is well, what's the rush? The option to wait and be monitored may not be presented to you, so you may have to ask for it, but in many cases it is a safe and sensible route to take.

You could take the view that there is no such thing as a 'late baby'. It's simply that some women naturally have a different length pregnancy than others. Regard those last few special days as a bonus. You can have a lie-in, read a book whenever you want, go out to a movie or for a meal at a whim. These are all things you will not be able to do again for a long time without a great deal of organisation, so enjoy them!

Membrane sweep

This will be written in your notes as 'sweep membranes', to take place at the first antenatal visit on or after your 'due date', or sometimes even before it. Your notes may simply say 'discuss membrane sweep', but a membrane sweep is so routine that it is assumed it will happen. It is such a routine procedure that it is hardly considered an intervention; but it is an intervention. And no intervention should be done without informed consent.

A membrane sweep consists of a midwife or obstetrician 'sweeping' a finger round the cervix during a vaginal examination to try to lift the membranes off the cervix. This can trigger the release of prostaglandins, which soften the cervix and can stimulate the onset of labour. To be thorough, a sweep should take about five minutes, and can be uncomfortable.

The reason that is often given for doing a sweep is, 'If we do a sweep today, it will save you from an induction next week, because baby will probably arrive quite quickly.' If you think for a moment, this is not a rational argument, because the baby will probably have arrived by next week anyway, and if it hasn't you could decide to have a sweep then. I have heard of women who had a sweep, went into labour, and had a very long labour, and then wondered afterwards if the baby would have arrived at the same time but with a shorter labour if they had left well alone.

Induction

About 20 per cent of labours in the UK are induced. The rate varies from country to country, but the percentage is high; much higher than the maximum of 10 per cent recommended by the World Health Organization. Consider this for a moment. For nine months your baby has grown perfectly normally. You go to antenatal visits to make sure all is well but, in general, everyone has assumed that the mother and baby know the best way to grow a baby. Then you get to the fictitious 'due date', which we have already seen is based on poor mathematics, and everyone knows better than that baby what it should be doing. How can it be that one in five mothers and babies have got it wrong?

Labour will not start until the cervix has softened, as the muscle needs to relax and release, so the first procedure in an induction is to apply prostaglandin gel to soften the cervix. This can cause uterine hyperstimulation, so you would probably be attached to a monitor, which is strapped to your abdomen, as your midwife or obstetrician will want to monitor your baby very carefully once you have received these powerful medications. This means you cannot move around freely and you cannot give birth in a birthing pool as you are attached to an electrical device, and because the staff are likely to want you to be on dry land in case any complications arise. It also means that you would have to be under the care of an obstetrician in a hospital obstetric unit, where more sophisticated emergency care is available. So you would be in a room with a bed and a chair, rather than at home or in a midwife-led unit (or birth centre), which is more likely to have rooms with birthing pools and birth balls, which generally encourage you to be in a position that could be more comfortable.

Usually synthetic oxytocin is also needed to stimulate surges, so the staff will insert a cannula, a small plastic tube (guided in with a needle which is then removed), usually in the mother's hand or arm. The cannula is attached to a bag of fluid containing the synthetic oxytocin, which further inhibits movement. Surges that are artificially stimulated tend to start more abruptly and be more frequent, more intense and closer together. In a natural labour, the muscles of the uterus revert to a resting state between surges. In an induced labour, the muscles remain in a low state of tension and never completely rest, so there is a greater strain on the mother's body and on the baby as the baby's oxygen supply is very slightly reduced compared with spontaneous labour.

An induced labour is a much more intense experience than a labour that starts naturally; it is more intense for the mother and more intense for the baby, so there is more likely to be foetal distress. However, I have known mothers do the whole of an induced labour without drugs using hypnobirthing techniques, which is a huge accolade for the mothers and for hypnobirthing – and also for her birth companion who is supporting her.

Two things can happen as a result of an induction. If the baby was almost ready to be born anyway, the labour can be intense but quite short. If the baby was not ready to be born or the mother is stressed and fearful, then the labour can be long, and there will come a point when she needs a rest. In order to rest she is given an epidural, a form of strong pain relief given through an injection in the back that numbs the lower half of the body.

An epidural is a sophisticated form of anaesthesia. It may numb your lower body, so not only does it block sensation from the lower part of your body to your brain, but also you can't feel the expulsive urges to birth your baby, and you may not be able to walk as you can't feel your legs. But you can have a light epidural (a walking epidural) which will have worn off before the second stage of labour and which allows you to walk. You can also have a self-administered epidural which you can top up yourself as needed but which also prevents you from overdosing.

A mother could also get a rest by having the synthetic oxytocin drip switched off, but I have never known this to happen. The effect of the epidural is to slow down her body and therefore possibly make labour longer. If it slows down her body, it can also slow down the baby's body. If the baby's heartbeat slows, it would be an indication for a Caesarean because the baby is in distress. If the mother's body slows down, she may need a top-up of synthetic oxytocin so that surges become even more powerful. Surges that are more powerful for the mother (although if her epidural is working well she may not be aware of this) are also more powerful for the baby, so the baby may become distressed and a Caesarean section is likely to be performed.

Because a heavy epidural block can result in a lack of sensation, the mother may not be able to feel when to bear down, so when her cervix is fully dilated she may need to be coached through the second stage rather than feeling her natural urge to expel her baby. This can mean that her body works less efficiently, and the birth is more likely to need a ventouse (vacuum extraction) or forceps intervention, or even a Caesarean. In her book *Breech Birth* (2003), the clinical psychologist Benna Waites tells us that the use of an epidural results in a three-times increase in instrumental delivery, a significant increase in the length of the second stage of labour (when the mother bears down and the baby is born), and double the Caesarean rate.

I would like to tell you a story that relates to inductions. When my fourth baby arrived I was going to have her at a small private hospital. I had no problem with the care I had received from the NHS; it was simply that during my pregnancy I had been looking after three little boys and I knew I was shortly going to be looking after three little boys and waking in the night to feed a new baby. So the concept of a room on my own for just a couple of days was extremely attractive.

My baby was due on 6 December, a Friday. At the end of November I went for an antenatal appointment, and after the usual checks there was a sharp drawing in of breath, a bit like a builder looking at a house, and I was told that I needed to be induced on 4 December. Jargon and phrases like 'fourth baby' and 'much safer for the baby' were thrown at me, and if somebody says to a mother it is safer for her baby, she will do anything. I pointed out that all my other babies had arrived two to four days so-called late, so plainly my natural length of pregnancy was about 40.5 weeks, which is perfectly normal. They said, 'No, it will be safer. We'll book you in for an induction on 4 December.'

So I went for my final antenatal visit on 2 December but in the interim all my sons had caught chickenpox. Other parents are generally quite prepared to look after children with chickenpox, since they would like their own children to get it, but not just before Christmas when granny is about to come to stay and everybody wants to be a happy family. It is almost impossible to find someone to look after three little boys with chickenpox just before Christmas. So I went to my last visit on 2 December saying, 'I don't think I can come to the induction on Wednesday because all my sons have chickenpox.' They looked at me in utter horror and said, 'Well, you can't have your baby here then.' A week before it had been very important that I should be induced on the 4th, and a week later I was almost unceremoniously kicked out into the gutter, because they were a small private hospital and if they had an epidemic they couldn't have taken people in, they would have lost income and their reputation would have plummeted. Maybe they would even have had to close.

I went back to the NHS hospital where I had had my other babies. They took me in, there was no mention of an induction, and my daughter was born without an induction on the Sunday afternoon, 8 December, so-called two days late just like her brothers. Better still, because of my sons' chickenpox, they put me in a little room on my own right at the end of the corridor, which I didn't have to pay for!

The real reason for the planned induction did not occur to me until I started to teach hypnobirthing. Then I received reports from lots of different midwife-led units and hospitals, and it gradually became clear that the only reason they wanted to induce me was to make sure my baby was not born at the weekend. It was the first weekend in December when there are lots of Christmas parties and people want to do their Christmas shopping. Maybe the consultant had a particular family gathering that he wanted to attend. Induce me on Wednesday, the baby is bound to have arrived by Friday, and everybody is happy – except mother and baby.

It is amazing the number of inductions that are done for convenience. It sounds very callous, but it is not, because any hospital has a maternity unit to run. They have to think of their staff. They have to manage everything for the overall good, and there will be a great many inductions just before Christmas and just before Easter. Maybe if a lot of mothers are booked in to give birth the following week they want to get through a few early so they can give the best possible care to everybody. Do bear this in mind and ask some questions if you are not quite sure why an induction is being suggested. You can find good information about inductions in the booklet 'Induction: Do I Really Need It?', which can be downloaded from the AIMS website, www.aims.org.uk.

Questions

When you hear the words 'allow', 'this is what we do' or 'we don't let you', I would suggest that you ask a few questions, because it is up to you whether you give consent, and you need information in order to do so. I'm not suggesting you simply tell a midwife or an obstetrician, 'No, I don't want that.' That would be rude and ill-informed; they have a great deal of knowledge and experience that should be respected. But it is your body and your baby, and you are entitled to be part of the decision-making process, which means you are also part of the dilemma that doctors and midwives face. Medical professionals face dilemmas daily. It is seldom that anything is black and white, that 'This is the right thing to do, and that is wrong.' It is more often a case of 'Taking everything into account, I think this would be a good option to try first' – bearing in mind that doing nothing can often be the best choice of all. No sensible person would object to any of the procedures suggested to help in certain medical circumstances. The problem arises when things are done routinely to every mother, sometimes without giving a full explanation to her, and without looking carefully at her individual circumstances, and taking her views into account.

The first question you might ask is '*I wonder if you can help me?*' It is a great question to use at the beginning of any conversation that could be difficult. Nobody would say, 'No.' They might not be able to say yes, but they will almost certainly say something like, 'I'll do my best', and then you're both on the same side at the start of the conversation, which is always the best place to be.

The next question, which is perfectly courteous and reasonable, is '*Could you explain that to me?*' It is even quite complimentary, because it recognises that the person is an expert. And they are an expert. But you are entitled to an explanation, and if you get a good explanation all other questions are superfluous. Sadly, though, sometimes you don't. I remember a woman expecting twins who asked me a question in a hypnobirthing class which was really a medical question, and I suggested she should ask her obstetrician. The answer her obstetrician gave was 'Because we think it's best', which is hardly a rational explanation to give to an intelligent adult. In fact, it's quite insulting.

In a situation like this you might need to ask some further questions. Never be rushed into making a decision. How often have you agreed to something, possibly as simple as going to see a movie one evening, then gone home and thought, 'I wish I hadn't agreed. I don't really want to see that film, and I would much rather stay at home and put my feet up.' Sometimes we rush into something and then regret it. And when it comes to your baby's birth, these are very important decisions. Always take your time. Say, 'Thank you for your advice, but we need a little time to think about what you've just told us.' Go home, sit down and have a cup of tea, sleep on it, discuss it with your husband, look it up on the Internet. And when you come to your own conclusion, based not only on the full facts and statistics, both for and against, but also on what your deepest instinct as a mother tells you is right, then let them know.

Another useful question is *'What other options are there that we could consider first?'* The staff in a busy maternity unit don't have time to explain everything to everybody, but if you ask, there are almost always other options, and you are entitled to be told about them and consider them.

You might like to ask *'How would what you're suggesting affect my labour* (or my wife or partner's labour)?' When I had my fourth baby I went into labour on a Sunday afternoon at about midday, and at four o'clock very little seemed to be happening and I was getting bored. My husband was even more bored. He was sitting on a stool beside me nodding off, so he went to the waiting room to find a more comfortable chair for a snooze. I remarked to the midwife that this labour was taking rather a long time. You might think that four hours is a reasonable length of time for a labour, but my first baby had arrived in six hours, my second in two hours, my third in half an hour, and so four hours was a rather unacceptable length of time as far as I was concerned.

The midwife was very sweet and told me, 'Baby would arrive quite quickly if I broke your waters.' Then, it being England and four in the afternoon, she asked, 'Would you like a cup of tea first?' So I had a cup of tea at 4pm, they broke my waters at 4.10pm, and baby arrived at 4.20pm. That quickly. It was a very hard and fast ten minutes, and I would never have agreed had I known. As it was my fourth baby it wasn't devastating, but had it been my first experience of childbirth it could have been. But nobody had said a word to explain the effects of the procedure, because it was so routine.

If we had asked how their suggestion would affect labour, just possibly somebody might have said that it would have been tougher. And of course, if it's more intense for the mother, it is also more intense for the baby; therefore, the question 'How would it affect the baby?' is also a very valid one.

If a particular procedure is proposed to avoid some possible negative outcome, it is worth asking 'Is it likely in this case?' Another very useful question is 'What will happen if we don't do this?' Most people go into hospital when they are ill, for something to be done, and so doing something tends to be the ethos of the hospital. But the option of not doing anything can be an extremely good one in many cases. So often, baby knows best.

You must respect the fact that there are, quite rightly, guidelines and protocols, and it is very difficult for a midwife to go against these protocols. She has to tick boxes. She will be in trouble if she does not, and her career might be put in jeopardy. It is quite right that there should be procedures for her to follow because, if there weren't guidelines, protocols and boxes to tick, things might get left out. However, remember that they should be guidelines, and not something that is followed religiously whatever the circumstances. Ask your midwife, '*Are you suggesting this because it's hospital protocol? In your personal opinion, is it best for me, and if so why?*' This gives her the space to talk around the issue and maybe a little more freely, rather than telling you simply, 'This is what we usually do.' In order not to tick the box, she has to be able to write 'mother declined', and you need a sensible discussion of the facts in order to make that decision.

It is also worth asking, '*Can you be sure that this will do more good than harm in my case?*' Of course, nobody can be absolutely sure of the outcome of an intervention, but if you can't be reasonably sure, why would you agree to it?

If you get really nervous you could say to the staff, '*Would you put that in writing please?*' You are required to sign that you agree to a procedure such as a Caesarean section, so it would seem reasonable to ask the obstetrician to sign the reason why a procedure is proposed.

I often hear reports of mothers being told things like 'Don't you want to do the best for your baby?' to get them to agree to a particular procedure. If you ask an obstetrician or midwife to put something in writing, they might possibly modify what they have been saying.

A useful mnemonic for decision-making is B-R-A-I-N:

Benefits
Risks
Alternatives
Instincts
Nothing

Each procedure has Benefits; each procedure has Risks – always. You are entitled to be told the benefits and risks in your case, and the statistics for when the procedure is or is not performed. Being told the risks of doing nothing and the benefits of what is proposed is not a full explanation. Both courses of action have benefits, and both have risks. You are entitled to know the research statistics for both.

There are always Alternatives, and if they haven't been presented to you then you need to ask. I am not saying that the alternatives are necessarily best, but to be told you have no choice is seldom an accurate assessment of the situation.

The 'I' stands for Instinct. A mother's instinct is powerful; it has ensured the continuation of the human race for millennia. If the mother's instinct says that something is or is not the right thing to do, then it should be treated with the greatest respect. 'I' can also stand for Information. Do you have enough information to make a sensible choice?

The last letter, 'N', is for Nothing. Nothing is a wonderful thing to do; it is much the best course of action until informed logic tells you that something else is an improvement.

I remember one mother I taught who went into labour very early. During the birth her husband suddenly said, 'I've got to get the questions', and rushed off to get them, because he felt he would support her better if he knew the right questions to ask, so you may find these questions very useful and they should be borne in mind seriously. In the event, this mother gave birth to a baby who weighed over 6lb, a perfectly normal size, so it seems that her natural length of pregnancy was less than the average 37–42 weeks: an example of a healthy baby of normal size being born outside the normal time parameters.

Remember that the law in the UK says no intervention may be done without informed consent. You may wish to remind your caregivers of this. Some things are done so routinely that they forget they are interventions. Once you have carefully taken advice and made your decision, any further discussion can be regarded as harassment.

Inducing labour more naturally

Some people try to bring on labour themselves to avoid a medical induction. But please remember that this is still a form of induction; it is still saying to your baby that you know better than he or she does when is the right time for their birth. Here is a list of things people do to bring on labour.

Lovemaking – Semen contains prostaglandin, which helps to soften the cervix, and when you make love you produce oxytocin, the hormone that stimulates uterine surges during labour. So there are two sound chemical reasons why making love is probably the best way to bring on labour. Also, making love relaxes you.

Nipple and clitoral stimulation – similar to lovemaking. Every midwife knows that this stimulation can help bring on labour, and some may suggest it, so to ask for privacy to do so at home or in the hospital is certainly not a strange request.

Laughter – relaxes you, and if a mother is relaxed she is more likely to go into labour. Have a small pile of funny or light-hearted DVDs at the ready.

Acupressure massage – see the illustrations opposite.
Spleen 6 (Sp 6) – find and rub this point on both your legs: four finger-widths up the calf from the top back 'corner' of the inside ankle bone.
Large Intestine 4 (LI 4) – this point is found on the side of the bone of your index finger, near the junction with your thumb. Press very firmly in towards the underside of the bone.

Hypnotherapy – the most effective of all the complementary therapies.

Homoeopathy, aromatherapy, reflexology, acupuncture, etc. – other complementary therapies that can be effective.

Visualising an opening rosebud – a soft and open image, which has a softening and opening effect on the body. Simple and surprisingly effective.

Walking – stimulates the blood's circulation to all the organs in the body, including the uterus. But don't get too tired.

Taking a bath – relaxes you.

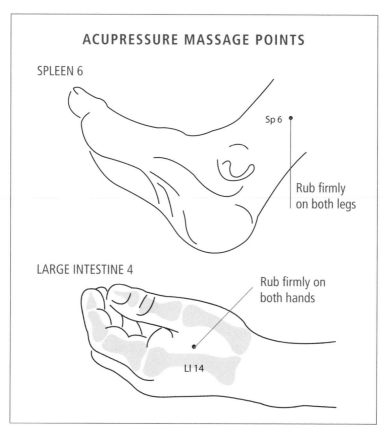

ACUPRESSURE MASSAGE POINTS

SPLEEN 6

Sp 6

Rub firmly on both legs

LARGE INTESTINE 4

Rub firmly on both hands

LI 14

Hot and spicy foods – Undoubtedly some women have gone into labour after a hot curry, but if it were that effective every woman in India would miscarry.

Raspberry leaf tea – a muscle toner not directly related to inducing labour, but because it tones muscles including the muscles of the uterus, it could stimulate them into action and so bring on labour.

Pineapple – has enzymes in it that may affect your hormones, but I have heard that you would have to eat about eight pineapples to have much of an effect.

Any of the above can trigger labour if you are nearly ready, but if you are nearly ready you will go into labour very soon anyway. I have heard mothers say they tried these things and labour started, but then it was a very long labour and perhaps the baby would have arrived at the same time but with a shorter labour if they had left well alone and waited for the baby to decide.

This is what a father told me afterwards about his wife having a membrane sweep and taking castor oil to bring on labour:

> I did read a lot about both practices, and although on the one hand I thought in principle they would interfere with the idea of a natural birth, on the other hand I thought they were pretty innocuous too: either they work or they don't.

He then went on to describe his wife's difficult labour and finished by saying:

> Patiently waiting is paramount; we knew that, you told us, we read it and told ourselves, and when it most

counted we ignored it all, thinking surely a 'little help' won't do any harm.

I would prefer that you never looked at the above list again, but I provide it because I am fairly sure you will. Mothers who have reached 40 weeks, and even before, drink raspberry leaf tea by the gallon. I would ask you to quietly consider why you are doing it and what is best for your baby.

If you are doing something to try to bring on labour, you are effectively saying to yourself that there is something wrong with the present situation. If you have decided there is something wrong, you have put yourself in a state of low-level stress. If you are in a state of stress, even at a low level, you are in the fear or emergency response, the sympathetic nervous system. As we saw in Chapter 2, you cannot be in the emergency response and the calm and confident response (the parasympathetic nervous system) at the same time. It is either one or the other. If you are in the calm and confident response, your body produces oxytocin, which is the hormone that stimulates the uterine muscles to work in labour, and therefore your baby is much more likely to put in an appearance. The body does not release when you are in a state of fear, even low-level stress, if it can possibly help it.

Objective medical advice

I strongly recommend that if you have a huge dilemma over a medical issue, it would be worth making an appointment with an independent midwife for some objective, experienced advice; just an hour or two will do. Go and see her or arrange for her to come to you and talk it through, and you will find that you definitely receive lots of good, objective information, and it will put your mind at rest. You can find a list of independent midwives at www.independentmidwives.org.uk.

CHAPTER 9

The Onset of Labour and Building Confidence

꧁꧂

'A mother's joy begins when new life is stirring inside … when a tiny heartbeat is heard for the very first time, and a playful kick reminds her that she is never alone.'

Anon.

The Onset of Labour and Building Confidence

There are a lot of theories but little conclusive evidence about what starts labour. One theory often put forward is that a mother goes into labour at the baby's instigation, when the baby releases a hormone into the mother's system, which triggers the mother's hormones, and after that it's a magical dance between the mother's and baby's hormones interplaying with each other.

T his happens when the baby is entirely ready for the world, when his or her little heart, lungs, kidneys, liver and brain are completely ready. Of course, the baby is often viable for several weeks before this, but it seems to be very presumptuous to think we know best, unless there is a particular indication that medical intervention is needed. It is known that there is considerable brain growth in the last few weeks of pregnancy, so it would seem wise to allow this to take place in its own time.

A show

One sign that labour can be starting is a 'show'. There is a mucous plug – mucous and slightly bloody – at the neck of the cervix, and a show is when it drops out because the cervix has begun to soften and open and doesn't hold it in any more. It may drop out into the loo so you don't notice it. Having a show doesn't necessarily mean your baby will be born immediately; it could happen a week before you go into labour.

Many women, however, particularly second-time mothers, would be found to be already 1cm dilated if they were examined a week before they went into labour. It doesn't mean they are in labour; it simply means the muscles have been practising.

Waters breaking

Another sign that labour is beginning is when a mother's waters break. This simply means that the amniotic sac, a bag of membranes, has released the amniotic fluid around the baby. The release of fluid is generally either a great gush or a steady flow of clear fluid, but it is not the same as a cervical weep, where there are only a few drops of clear, odourless fluid and which can happen days, or even a week or two, before labour starts. If the membranes release, it is likely that you will go into labour quite soon; most women will go into labour within 24 hours.

The purpose of the membranes and the amniotic fluid around the baby is that they protect him or her from physical trauma, so if you forget how big you are and bang into a doorpost, your baby will be fine because of this protection.

The fluid also keeps the baby at a fairly even temperature. So if you are pregnant in Rio in the summer and the temperature is 40°C, your baby will stay comfortably cool. If you are pregnant in Alaska in the winter where it's −30°C, the fluid will keep your baby perfectly warm.

Inhaling and exhaling the fluid helps your baby's lungs to develop.

The bag of membranes also keeps the baby free from infection. As soon as the membranes have released, this is no longer the case, but your body does still continue to make amniotic fluid, which will continue to be released downwards, washing possible infections away from your baby.

For this reason it makes sense to have no internal examinations after the waters release, as each one increases the chance that an infection such as Group B Streptococcus (GBS) may be introduced higher up inside you, putting your baby at a greater risk of infection.

GBS is an infection that occurs quite frequently. Probably 20 to 30 per cent of women would have it if you took a swab of the vagina at any time. You could take another swab a month later and it might not be present, or vice versa, which is why some countries do not test for Group B Streptococcus because it is transient and not doing any harm to the mother. But in very rare cases it can do harm to a newborn baby. It is a meningitis-type infection and can cause brain damage or death, though this is very rare. The vast majority of babies born to mothers after their waters have released for an extended time are absolutely fine and healthy.

If your waters break and you have not gone into labour within 24 hours, it is very likely that you will be strongly advised to have an induction. You will also be put on a drip of antibiotics to deal with infection, most importantly GBS. There are arguments for and against these procedures, and again you have choices. In such a situation you need to ask, 'What are the risks of having an induced labour?' and 'What are the risks of Group B Streptococcus?' Ask lots of questions and ask for statistics. Then you can sensibly weigh up the risks and benefits against each other and make your decision. Make sure you feel comfortable with what you decide.

The problem with antibiotics is that they greatly reduce the benign bacteria as well as the harmful bacteria. The immune system is largely modulated in the gut, and if you destroy the bacteria in the mother's gut you weaken her immune system. In the rare event that antibiotics are justified, it is very important for the mother to take good-quality probiotics afterwards to reinoculate the gut, otherwise the gut may become colonised by any opportunistic bacteria. I am delighted to say that recently I have heard of two hospitals that do provide probiotics after the administration of antibiotics, which is an encouraging step.

Here is an excerpt from an article in *Mothering* magazine (2003) about GBS and the effect of antibiotics, given to the mother during labour, on newborn babies:

> *Some studies have shown a decrease in GBS infection in newborns whose mothers accepted intravenous (IV) antibiotics during labour, but no decrease in the incidence of death. Still other research has found that preventative use of antibiotics is not always effective. In fact, one study found no decrease in GBS infection or deaths in newborns whose mothers were given IV antibiotics during labour.*
>
> *Perhaps the greatest area of concern to medical researchers, as it should be to us all, is the alarming increase in antibiotic-resistant strains of bacteria. Antibiotic-resistant bacteria can cause infections in newborns that are very difficult to treat. Many large research studies have found not only resistant strains of GBS, but also antibiotic-resistant strains of E. coli and other bacteria caused by the use of antibiotics in labouring women. Some strains of GBS have been found to be resistant to treatment by all currently used forms of antibiotics.*
>
> *While many studies have found that giving antibiotics during labour to women who test positive for GBS decreases the rate of GBS infection among newborns, research is beginning to show that this benefit is being outweighed*

*by increases in other forms of infection. One study, which
looked at the rates of blood infection among newborns
over a period of six years, found that the use of antibiotics
during labour reduced the incidence of GBS infection in
newborns but increased the incidence of other forms of
blood infection. The overall effect was that the incidence
of newborn blood infection remained unchanged.*

So, as you can see, there are no easy answers, and if anything is presented to you as being the only course of action that is safe for your baby, it really isn't that simple. Some mothers feel more comfortable taking antibiotics while others prefer to wait. I have known mothers wait anything up to seven days and have their baby normally and in good health. Yes, there are risks, but the risks are not all on one side. We know there are risks and benefits to both courses of action. In many cases, nature knows best, but occasionally we can be grateful for help.

Surges (contractions or uterine waves)

The most usual way of going into labour is when tightenings start in your abdomen. Probably in late pregnancy the muscles of your abdomen have been tightening from time to time. Sometimes they go really hard, and then slacken off. The more you progress in pregnancy, the more often these waves of activity of the uterine muscles happen, and then one day the surges seem to come quite frequently and become more regular, and you begin to time it, and the tightening comes every half hour, then every 20 minutes, then 15 minutes, then every 25 minutes … And then it stops, just when you thought your baby really was on its way. A couple of days later exactly the same thing happens, but this time it goes on and it really is the beginning of your baby's arrival in the world.

But the contractions can begin in a completely different way, because everyone is different. I have known mothers who were not quite sure if labour had started or not, then the baby arrived. Another mother went out with her husband to see a movie and have a meal in a restaurant about a week before her baby was due. She came home, lay down in bed, and instantly her surges started, five minutes apart and one minute long, five minutes apart and one minute long, on and on. The rhythm never varied throughout the whole of her labour, so she knew exactly when her labour started; there was no doubt about it at all.

But more often than not you are not quite sure if your baby is really coming, or if it isn't, or perhaps it is; perhaps we ought to call the midwife; no, it's not really worth it just yet – you are not sure if labour has started or not. Always wait until you are absolutely sure, for as long as you possibly can, before calling the midwife or going into hospital, because so often labour can slow down if you go into hospital too early.

Useful phrases

I'll tell you now Mary Cronk's useful phrases. Mary is a highly respected midwife (now retired) to whom many midwives and mothers have turned for advice over the years, particularly with regard to her knowledge and experience of breech babies and twins being born at home. This was her advice to the mothers in her care:

I am sure many others will explain your absolute right to refuse any procedure for any or no reason. The law and good practice are quite clear. A sensible person will listen carefully to any explanations as to why a procedure is proposed, and then should she choose not to have X, Y or Z she just says 'No' or 'No, thank you'. The 'allowing' is done by YOU. An assertive approach is worth cultivating. The following phrases have been found useful by women encountering difficulties, and are in order of assertiveness. You may care to commit them to memory and practise them frequently (three times a day) in front of a mirror.

1 'Thank you so much for your advice, which I/we will consider carefully and let you know my/our decision.' *Sweet smile! This phrase is most useful in the antenatal stage, but it can be used in labour. It can take a little while to consider either what you want to know, or what you decide.*

2 'Would you like to repeat what you just said?' *(spoken in a voice of incredulity). This is useful and, for example, applies to the misuse of the word 'allow'.*

3 'I'm afraid I shall have to regard any further discussion as harassment' *(said with a look of sorrow). This can be said if a person does not respect your decision or persists in pressing the subject.*

4 'Don't you think you're being rather impertinent?'

5 'What is your NMC PIN number?' *(To a nurse or midwife, who must be registered with the Nursing & Midwifery Council to be able to work in the UK.)* What is your GMC PIN number?' *(To a medical practitioner, who must be registered with the General Medical Council.) This can be used if the above phrase is ineffective. If the person asks why you want their PIN number, inform them that this is something they might like to consider.*

6 *To be used* in extremis: 'Stop this AT ONCE.' *I am delighted to tell you that this was used against me by a*

woman to whom I had taught it to. I was doing a difficult
vaginal examination and was being too persistent. I stopped
at once and learnt a lesson.

You can always leave – or tell the person involved to leave.
Get out before bursting into tears. Remember you are going
to be someone's parent, a position of great importance and
responsibility. You are not a weak and feeble woman. You
are strong and powerful.
Please do not be drawn into 'fighting'. Just state your
intentions clearly and calmly. Do not argue, but learn these
phrases, or similar ones, and keep them for use if necessary.
I am informed it is usually only necessary to be assertive
once or twice to have a much more respectful attitude from
the people who are actually your professional servants.

(Thank you, Mary, for permission to use these words.)

Releasing fears and building confidence

Here is an important exercise for you to do. Write a list of
everything that concerns you or worries you about birth:
having a baby, what your mother-in-law is going to say,
how expensive it is going to be, or absolutely anything that
comes to mind which you consider worrying about birth.
If something comes to mind that doesn't seem to be related,
put it down anyway, because if you are thinking of it now, it
may come to mind while you are giving birth to your baby.
It's very useful to allow fears that might have been quite deep
down to come to the surface and be written down. When
they are out there on a piece of paper, it stops them buzzing
around your head and helps to take away their power. Ask
your husband or partner to write a list, too. Make your lists
separately, as this is an individual process.

Now compare your lists. However much we know and love the person we live with, we may not be aware of something that is really worrying them, and we might be able to help if we did know. On the other hand, we might think that something is a concern to them, and desperately try to protect them, when actually it is not something that worries them at all. So compare your notes, and then read the following script to release those fears, which is an important part of hypnobirthing. Read the script to each other, or get the CD *Confidence and Power* (see the back of the book) and listen to it together.

CONFIDENCE AND POWER

Sit back and relax. Now let your eyes close, slowly and gently. Just relax ... relax ... relax. Notice your breathing, how soft and quiet it has become, as you relax even further.

Now you may begin to feel just as relaxed throughout your entire body, so you allow a wave of warmth and contentment to wash all through you, starting at the very top of your head as a gentle, warm, golden light that penetrates softly every part of you. Slowly it moves down through your head: your eyelids, all around your eyes, your cheeks, your lips, your jaws, everything calms and relaxes. Just let that feeling spread on down through your neck, your shoulders, and down your arms. It flows down into your chest, through your stomach, your pelvis, all the way down your upper legs, your knees, your lower legs, your feet, until it reaches your toes, and every single part of your body is completely relaxed in this gentle, golden glow.

Everything around you helps you to relax more and more deeply: your breathing, the music, my voice, and even if an unexpected sound breaks in, like a car passing, or voices outside, or a phone ringing, that sound will simply be a trigger to allow you to relax even more.

Just as you think you are as deeply relaxed as you can be, you begin to relax even more deeply.

Now, just imagine yourself in a lift on the tenth floor of a building. This is a very good, comfortable, safe lift, and completely smooth and silent, and you press the button to begin to take you all the way down. As the lift moves, you watch the lights for the different floors. Ten ... the lift has just started on its way down. Nine ... you find yourself going deeper into relaxation as the lift descends, going deeper with it. Eight ... as you see the number light up, you go further into yourself. Seven ... your whole body starts to feel completely weightless. Six ... you are floating on a wave of relaxation as if on a soft cloud. Five... deeper, deeper still. Four ... you have entered your own true self, deeply and willingly. Three ... you are so focused within your whole being that nothing touches you but your own true self, your wisdom, your intuition. Two... everything is slipping away but your mind and your thoughts. One ... you feel completely, deeply and wonderfully relaxed, free of all care and worries, happy and peaceful. Even your thoughts are fading into oblivion. So deep; so very, very deep.

Rest, just rest happy and relaxed for a while. There's plenty of time.

Now imagine a blue-skied summer's day and you are lying on soft, dry grass under a tree by the sea. A warm, gentle

Continued overleaf...

... Continued from page 143

breeze just lightly touches your cheek. You are completely serene, happy and peaceful.

As you look up, you notice that the leaves of the tree have pictures of all your happy memories, but also a few of them have images of the upsetting things in your life that make you wonder about giving birth. As you look at the leaves you notice some images that bring to mind things you have heard or read or thought about the concerns of childbirth, or your own previous experience of giving birth. As you observe and study the first one, you notice that the image gradually fades into the leaf itself, which then turns yellow, brown, then gold – the colours of autumn – meaning the leaf has come to the end of its time, and neither it nor the thought it held matter any longer; and then the leaf just drops off the tree and lands beneath it.

Now you notice another leaf with another concern and it too gently fades and dissolves into the leaf, which changes colour and flutters to the ground, joining the first one.

As you look, each time a concern you have comes to mind, a leaf takes on that image, which then fades and disappears as the leaf changes colour and falls to earth.

You realise now that you are able to see all these concerns in the leaves, so you just take all the time you need to make sure all are dealt with – concerns about birth, or anything else that comes to mind and which you would like to easily release. You find that one by one the same thing happens. The image of each concern is taken on by a leaf, and is absorbed into the leaf, until it completely disappears. And all the leaves concerned change colour through the shades of autumn – yellow, brown, gold – and flutter to earth, taking their now vanished concerns with them, and when the process is complete you sweep the leaves up into a heap.

Now only happy and joyful green leaves are left on the tree and as you wonder what to do with the pile of leaves beside you, you have an idea. You decide you will have a bonfire, and invite to it all the people who have helped you in the past or who are helping you now, or who are going to help you at this wonderful and important time in your life. Soon they start to arrive. They all come. You and your partner are both there of course, your mother and father, other family members, friends from throughout your life including right back to school, perhaps some of the people who taught you, your midwife, your doctor, employers, colleagues, just everyone who has ever helped or supported you, and those who will support you during the rest of your pregnancy and your baby's birth.

When they have all arrived and you are one big, happy gathering, you set light to the bonfire. It blazes quickly, and the leaves that had all the upsetting memories start to burn and curl up in the crackling flames. As they curl up and burn they turn to ash, and the ash rises in the heat, and as it rises, the gentle breeze picks it up and wafts it out to sea. You watch the ash as it floats further and further out over the water until it completely vanishes from sight. And as it vanishes completely, those memories and feelings the leaves carried vanish completely with it, gone forever, leaving you so confident and calm, peaceful and happy.

You feel so confident as you realise that you now completely accept yourself and your intuitive power to control your own life and look after yourself and your baby. Although all these people have helped, or are helping or will help you, you now see that, while you accept their help, gladly and gratefully, you remain in control of your own life, and you and only you decide how things are to be, and how these people may help you so

Continued overleaf...

... Continued from page 145

that your baby is born so easily and happily, entering the world in the best possible way and giving you an empowering and joyful experience. And with this wonderful self-confidence and happiness, your guests slowly fade away, and leave you to your new self, knowing you can call them whenever you want them, and feeling confident that you will know when and how you need their wisdom, experience and knowledge to help you.

These thoughts lead you to realise that you can decide how you want the birth of your baby to be. You decide how your labour is, and just how short a time it takes. Take a little while now to choose ... Consider too how comfortable it will be, how calm and relaxed. Remember that your body is created to give birth gently and naturally, and at the right time and place, to allow your baby's easy and serene passage into the world, so that you can for the first time hold your beautiful baby in your arms. You realise now that it's easy to decide all these things in your new confidence; and the power that gives you, and the happiness and calmness it brings you, allow you to drift deeper into peace and calmness, confidence and wellbeing.

Now you look up with gratitude to the tree with all its green leaves with their happy memories, and something wonderful happens. The leaves separate and form a beautiful green picture frame, and the picture inside that frame is you, both of you, with your baby in your arms. You look so happy and radiant, knowing that all happened just as you had visualised it. Your baby is sleeping gently in the crook of your arm, so sweet and gentle and secure. You are filled with love and happiness.

The picture seems to float gently down from the tree and it becomes life-size as it envelops you, and now, like a miracle, you realise that this is not a picture at all. It is real, and what seemed to be a picture of you both with your baby now really is you, and you feel overjoyed at your success. A feeling of such gentle tenderness comes over you as you look down at your baby's face and it opens its eyes and looks into yours. All is so perfectly as you planned it to be, and you will remember this feeling over and over again until the day when it really happens.

So in a minute it will be time to return to everyday reality, but a different reality, as you remember all you have just experienced and the joy it gave you and will continue to give you, as your pregnancy progresses, as you give birth to your baby, and after your baby is born.

As I count from five to one, gently and gradually come back to the present. Five ... feeling the weight returning to your body. Four ... gently feeling tiny movements in your fingers and toes. Three ... your eyelids begin to feel lighter. Two ... you feel alert and calm, happy and relaxed. One ... your eyes open as you quietly and gently rejoin me in this room in calm confidence.

Now that you have released your fears, never look at your lists again. You have dealt with the concerns. This is one piece of paper that you do not recycle. Tear it up, shred it, burn it. Destroy it utterly and never look at it again.

This is not a relaxation and release for everyday practice, but use it if something happens that gives you a major wobble; maybe you hear a very negative birth story, or something happens that you hadn't foreseen. Take out this script and use it again, so you can deal with that circumstance, or anything else that may arise.

CHAPTER 10

The Up Stage
of Labour

*'We find a delight in the beauty and
happiness of children, that makes
the heart too big for the body.'*

Ralph Waldo Emerson,
The Conduct of Life, 1860

The Up Stage of Labour

In the first stage of labour, as we saw earlier, the upper muscles of the uterus are working to draw up, which is why I call it the 'up' stage of labour. At the same time the internal muscles in the lower uterus around the cervix release, so these muscles become thinner and draw back until the cervix is fully open. Then the uterus works in a downward direction to birth the baby; this is called the second or 'down' stage of labour.

Early labour

In early labour, gently keep doing whatever you feel like. You can continue whatever you were doing before labour began, or anything at all as long as it is gentle. You can have a rest, or read one of the relaxation scripts if that would be helpful. Most of the work of the scripts is done before labour, but some people find it useful to read one in early labour as well. You can watch one of your funny DVDs. That's what they're for: to relax the body and mind in early labour. You can put on the *Colour and Calmness* CD or have the script read to you, because you're used to relaxing to the sound, and so is your baby. It is amazing the number of mothers who have told me they did the ironing in early labour – mothers who are not noted for being addicted to ironing. Maybe it's the rhythm and the warmth; I don't know.

It is important to conserve energy, because however gentle your labour, you will need your energy later on. You will get a little adrenaline surge just before you go into labour, and if that stimulates your nesting instincts to sort through all the baby clothes, that's fine. But if you start moving all the furniture in the house – fathers, stop her! Mothers need their energy for the later stages of labour. I've heard of plenty of mothers who have walked when labour appeared to be starting to try and 'get things going' and then wished they hadn't afterwards when they realised they had wasted energy.

It's a good idea to snack, so do raid the fridge. I'm not saying have a ten-course dinner, but have a light snack now and again if you feel like it, to keep your energy up. Also drink water, but I don't mean drink gallons. When I had my first baby I was told to drink water, so I drank copiously with the result that, when I was in established labour, I kept rushing backwards and forwards to the loo. Fathers, make sure she has a jug of water beside her, and pour out a glass so she can sip it now and again. If she hasn't had any water for a couple of hours, just suggest quietly that it might be an idea to have a sip.

There will come a time when you may find the up breathing that you learnt in Chapter 3 useful. It helps to relax and calm you. The up visualisations that you learnt with this breathing ensure that mind and body are working together, so you may find it helpful to bring them to mind, or else have your birth companion gently remind you of them during surges. Or you may prefer silence.

Movies portray labour as an emergency, with people rushing about and blue flashing lights on ambulances. It isn't an emergency. It is a quiet time for you to go gently further and further into yourself. There is plenty of time. Just because a woman is having a baby, it doesn't mean that she doesn't know if she is thirsty or wants a rest. In fact, her intuitive awareness of her needs and the needs of her baby are much heightened and should be treated with the greatest respect.

You are usually told to go into hospital or to call the midwife to come to you when the tightenings are about four minutes apart and one minute long. Definitely go to hospital later rather than sooner. First-time mothers tend to go into hospital far too soon.

It is usually the father who makes the call and the person on the other end will say, 'Can I speak to her?' Hypnobirthing mothers are usually calm and therefore the person can be confused and think she is not in established labour. There are several ways of dealing with this. The father can say, 'She can't possibly come to the phone.' Or you can take the phone and do some pretend heavy breathing. Or you can tell them that you're doing hypnobirthing. These days people are more used to hypnobirthing and they will hopefully understand that mothers doing hypnobirthing can be in very well-established labour but still remain calm and have a perfectly coherent conversation.

Sometimes if you're planning a homebirth, they will say they are too busy to send a midwife so you will have to come into the unit. Note the phrase 'You will have to.' When you think about this for a minute, that is the time you particularly don't want to be in the unit because, if they are so busy, each midwife may be looking after two or three mothers. They will be extremely rushed and you will certainly not get one-to-one care. If you stay at home you will get one-to-one care, because an experienced midwife is sent out just for you.

Homebirth

It is generally agreed that one-to-one care during labour from a known and trusted midwife makes a profound difference to the experience and outcome of labour. Sadly, in most hospitals these days you don't get this care, because the staff are too busy and there is a shortage of midwives. One way of getting one-to-one care on the NHS is to have your baby at home, because a midwife is sent out just for you. She will probably be an experienced midwife, because she is sent out to you on her own. A second midwife will arrive to assist her in late labour, in time for the birth.

If you decide to have your baby at home, you will have exactly the same technical support as you have in a midwife-led unit (or birth centre). You have the same support in terms of pain relief. You have gas and air, and either the midwife will provide pethidine or you can get it on prescription from your doctor in advance. You have the same equipment in terms of resuscitation for the baby: oxygen is brought and masks for the baby and the mother. The midwife will also have the injection to use in the rare event of haemorrhage. She will also have equipment to monitor the baby's heart rate.

Of course there is more technical support in a hospital, where they offer epidurals, ventouse and forceps deliveries and Caesarean sections. But most people go to a midwife-led unit, because that is where you get the home-from-home rooms and the birthing pools. Why do they make the rooms more like home? Because a mother feels more relaxed in a home environment and so labour progresses more smoothly. If you have your baby at home, you are in your own environment and you have everything there that makes you feel comfortable and at ease. And you can sleep in your own bed afterwards. So you get everything that you would get in a midwife-led unit, plus the huge advantage of one-to-one care.

People often worry about transferring from home to hospital, the 'what ifs'. They have an image of blue flashing-light emergencies. There are risks at homebirths; there are risks at hospital births. The risks are different, and they are tiny, and home and hospital are equally safe for most mothers. One of the main risks of a hospital birth is infection; there are superbugs that can be very difficult to treat, which would not be a threat at home. The two most common reasons for transfer from home to hospital are failure to progress (by definition not an emergency) or because there is meconium in the amniotic fluid. I spoke to a very experienced homebirth midwife recently who had only one emergency transfer in five years.

Meconium is the sticky black substance that a baby passes in the first few days of life before its stools becomes soft and yellow. The presence of meconium in the amniotic fluid means the baby has had a bowel movement before or during labour, which could mean the baby is in distress. The guidelines these days are that, if the amniotic fluid is clear, all is well; if the amniotic fluid is a brownish colour but there are no lumps in it, all is well; but if there are lumps of meconium in the amniotic fluid, there is a risk of the baby inhaling a lump, which could inhibit breathing, so it makes sense to be in hospital where more sophisticated resuscitation equipment is available. Lumps of meconium are not an immediate risk in labour because the baby is still receiving oxygen through the cord from its mother, but they would become a risk factor if they cause obstruction of the airways when the baby starts to breathe for itself after birth.

If you have a homebirth you have a midwife one-to-one just for you and so, if there should be a reason for transfer, she will pick it up quickly. She will summon an ambulance or ask your husband or partner to do this. She may travel in the ambulance with you or she may travel in her car, with your partner following in your car with your bags and baby car seat ready for coming home later. She will have called ahead to tell the hospital that you are coming and why, and when you get there, the team will be ready to deal with whatever the reason was for the transfer.

If you are in a hospital, there may not be a midwife with you all the time, so it might be 15 or 20 minutes before she comes into the room and picks up if there is anything that should be done in the event of something unusual happening. She will then have to call for support and muster the team, which will take 10 or 15 minutes, so it could take as long, or possibly even longer, to get support if you are in a hospital or birth centre than if you are at home.

The statistics for transfer from homebirth for first babies is roughly 40 per cent and very much less for those having a second or subsequent baby, and the majority of those transfers is because of failure to progress. This means that 60 per cent of first-time homebirths and more like 95 per cent of second or subsequent births take place normally and naturally. If you look at the statistics for hospital births conducted normally and naturally, without intervention, the numbers are much lower. If you transfer to hospital in labour, it is only what you would have done anyway if you had at first planned to give birth in hospital. All these facts are worth thinking about.

If you are having your baby at home, it is very helpful to your midwife for you to make it obvious which is your house. It doesn't matter if she knocks on the wrong door at 3pm, but it matters very much at 3am. Midwives have been known to go up and down the road (or the staircases in flats) if the right house is not apparent, so have an agreed sign such as having all the lights on or a balloon on the door to make it easy for her.

It is interesting to note that in 1992 a House of Commons investigation concluded that, 'On the basis of what we have heard, this Committee must draw the conclusion that the policy of encouraging all women to give birth in hospitals cannot be justified on grounds of safety.'

Travelling to hospital

If you are travelling to hospital by car, labour can slow down or even reverse, so wait until you are in well-established labour. Many mothers feel they are in well-established labour and go to hospital, only to be told they are only 1cm dilated and sent home again. I often wonder how many of these mothers really were in established labour when they were at home, but it was the unnatural experience of leaving the safety of their home, travelling in a car, and going to a strange place to be examined by strangers (however kind) that actually made the whole process reverse. We shall never know, but it is certainly something that the female of no other species would do.

If you transfer, it can be more comfortable kneeling on the back seat of the car with your head down (in yoga terms, the pose of the child) rather than sitting in the front seat with your seat belt on. Just do what is most comfortable.

Hospital

If you are going to an obstetric unit or a birth centre to have your baby, it can be nice to take things with you to make it as much like home as possible. You might take a pillow, or some clothing from your husband or older child, or a photo from your bedside table; anything that makes the room feel more like home. Smell is a very basic animal sense, and it can make a big difference to how you settle into a new environment.

When you get to the hospital, you have the process of triage (checking in), which can take some time if they are busy. You may have the impression from your antenatal hospital tour that you arrive at the hospital and are instantly ushered into your lovely room. This depends on how busy they are. You may find you are sitting (or sometimes standing) waiting for quite some time. So just practise your up breathing and do your visualisations, as you do in hypnobirthing throughout the up (first) stage of labour.

Birthing pools

Many mothers have found that giving birth in water is relaxing and comforting. I have heard it said that the effect of a birthing pool is as good as an injection of pethidine – and with no harmful effects.

If you are having your baby at home, you can hire or buy a birthing pool. If you hire a pool, you will need to hire it from about week 37 in case your pregnancy is shorter than average, and possibly keep it until week 43 in case your pregnancy is longer. You can choose a solid one with a heater and a lid so that you can fill it in advance and use it to relax in before your baby is born. If you buy a birthing pool, an inflatable pool is the cheapest option and is perfectly adequate. They come in two sizes, and the smaller size will be big enough. You might be able to buy a pool through eBay, in which case you just need to buy a new polythene liner for it, and you can resell the pool on eBay afterwards or donate it to your local homebirth group or independent midwife, who will make good use of it for other mothers. Sometimes it is possible to borrow one from your local homebirth group so you don't have to buy one at all.

It is a very good idea to have a practice run setting up the pool before your baby is born, to ensure everything is there and working well, and that you know how to do it. You want to be sure, for instance, that the tap fitting works on your taps. Pools come with a pump and a hose so you don't have to take ages filling them with bowls of water. Every midwife-led unit in the UK has a birthing pool, and hospitals are beginning to install them too, because mothers who need extra support in labour will also benefit from the extra comfort of labouring in a birthing pool. It is gloriously relaxing.

You are usually told not to get into the pool until you are 5cm dilated. It is another occasion when the phrase 'You are not allowed' is often used; a phrase which should set off alarm bells in your head. The reason for this advice is that you might relax so much that labour slows down, and I have heard of this happening in a couple of cases. Usually the comfort of the warm water allows any tension you are holding in your body to drop away and labour progresses more quickly. If labour did slow down because you were in the pool, I am sure you would have the intelligence to get out if that was suggested to you.

The funny thing is that mothers who ring the hospital too early in labour are often told to go and have a nice, warm bath and relax. As soon as they get into hospital in established labour, they are told they are not allowed to get into the warm, comfortable birthing pool because it slows labour down. An interesting anomaly.

Vaginal examinations

Internal examinations are routinely done when you first get to hospital to see how far dilated your cervix is; to check if you are 5cm dilated before you are 'allowed' to get into a birthing pool; and to see if you are fully dilated – that your cervix is about 10cm dilated – before you are 'allowed' to push.

Many midwives – many independent midwives – will have the experience to support you in labour safely, gently and extremely well without doing any vaginal examinations. In many cases, most cases indeed, you are absolutely fine without them. No woman likes to have a vaginal examination. The more experienced the midwife, the less she will rely on them. A vaginal examination simply tells her how far dilated you are at that moment. It does not tell her how, or how fast, labour will progress. There may be a particular circumstance where a midwife would find the information gained useful, in which case, if this was explained to you, I am sure you would agree to an examination. But just because something is usually done, it doesn't necessarily mean that it is in your best interests. A mother I spoke to recently had been having mild surges (pre-labour) for two days, and then progressed from 2cm dilated to fully dilated in 10 minutes. It is equally possible that a woman could reach 7cm dilation in a couple of hours, and then everything slows down for a while. Another mother told me recently how she had two babies without a single vaginal examination at any time – two very quick and straightforward births. I wonder if the two facts could be connected?

Remember also that, as we saw in the previous chapter, after your waters break each internal examination increases the chance of introducing infections inside you, so it makes sense to avoid examinations in these circumstances to help protect your baby from infection.

Rapport with your midwife

Another thing I would like to talk about is communication with your midwife. Midwives are lovely people, but they are not necessarily psychic, and so if you don't tell them you are doing hypnobirthing, how are they to know? They want to support you, and they wouldn't be in the profession if they didn't: the hours are appalling and the pay is not that amazing, but when you're present at the miracle of a birth, there is nothing like it.

So I would suggest you write a little note to the midwife. You've probably done a longer birth plan as well, but that might be tucked away in your notes and there may not be a lot of time for the staff to study it closely if the unit is busy. So write a very short note, preferably in your own handwriting and your own words. Take several copies with you in case there is a shift change, so your partner can give a copy to anyone who comes into the room and then everyone knows what you are doing. I would suggest it says something like this:

We have been practising hypnobirthing and our focus is on a calm and natural birth. We would very much appreciate your support in this by helping us to create a calm and quiet environment at all times, both physically, mentally and emotionally, with no interventions and no vaginal examinations without our fully informed consent and unless absolutely necessary. We would particularly request that no coaching is given during the second stage of labour and that all conversation is kept to the absolute minimum.

If you have any questions, please ask my husband (or insert the name of your birth companion) *in the first instance, and not me.*

Thank you so much for your help.

Let's go through it. '*We have been practising hypnobirthing and our focus is on a calm and natural birth.*' Now the midwife knows what you are doing. Almost every woman in pregnancy will say, 'I want a natural birth; I don't like drugs', but the minute she arrives at hospital she asks for an epidural. Midwives have seen this time and time again. The difference between this and a hypnobirthing mother is that you have done something to achieve a natural birth and you are very likely to get it. More and more midwives are now beginning to have experience of hypnobirthing, and they know very well that if you have done hypnobirthing, you are very likely to achieve what you want – a natural birth for you and your baby. Tell her what you have been doing and she will be in a better position to support you.

'*We would very much appreciate your support in this.*' Your midwife wants to support you, so ask for her help – so that everybody is working together.

'*… By helping us to create a calm and quiet environment at all times, both physically, mentally and emotionally.*' People may understand about quiet rooms, low music and soft lights, but mental and emotional quietness are even more important, and unguarded words can create enormous stress. So it is a good idea to remind your midwife of the importance of this right at the beginning. It is also very helpful if your husband, partner or birthing companion knows about hypnobirthing, though many women use hypnobirthing extremely effectively without such support.

'*No interventions and no vaginal examinations without our fully informed consent unless absolutely necessary.*' I would like to reiterate that I am always talking about a normal, natural situation, and that I am not medically qualified. I am certainly not suggesting you disregard medical advice. However, as we have seen in earlier chapters, many things are done absolutely routinely and mothers say afterwards, 'If I had known I would never have agreed.' It is a different way round if you start from the premise that you are not going to have anything done unless it is fully explained to you and there is a particular medical need, rather than from the assumption that you will have all the routine procedures. It makes for a gentler and more natural labour.

Please note the above phrase does not say you have declined all interventions. It simply says that the starting point is that nothing will be done, but if a particular course of action is fully explained to you, then you will consider whether to give your consent. The law says that no procedure may be done without informed consent. Information does not mean someone telling you why they think it is a good idea. It means that all the risks and benefits of the proposed procedure, plus all the risks and benefits of an alternative course of action (remember that everything has benefits and everything has risks), are fully explained to you, together with the statistical likelihood of each if you were to find that useful.

'*We would particularly request that no coaching is given during the second stage of labour and that all conversation is kept to the absolute minimum.*' Why is it that, for the most part, it is assumed that a mother knows how to grow and birth her baby, until it comes to the point when she is ready to ease her baby down the birth canal, and then she needs to be coached? This is completely unnecessary for a hypnobirthing mother, and even distracting, and therefore it can be harmful. After the baby is born, too, it is the most special moment, and conversation from the midwife is superfluous and intrusive.

'*If you have any questions, please ask my husband* (or insert the name of your birth companion) *in the first instance, and not me.*' This little message has to come from you, the mother, because legally you are the patient and therefore instructions can only be taken from you. Of course, the midwife will also look to your partner to tell her what you want so as not to disturb you, but this phrase allows her to do that. If something is put in writing, it should be in terms that are helpful to her.

Adding this message doesn't mean that decisions are taken by your husband or partner for you. It simply means that any run-of-the-mill questions can pass you by. When you start answering questions, the thinking part of your brain clicks into gear and, as we've seen, it is activity in that part of the brain that flips you from the confident state into the fear response. So the fewer questions and the less that you are bothered, the better.

I remember a mother who did hypnobirthing, and who told me that she was in a birthing pool at home when her baby's heartbeat began to slow just a little. This is something that you must take very seriously. The midwife said to the father in the kitchen, 'I think we should transfer to the hospital.' The father talked it through with the midwife. He asked if it was an emergency or if it would be safe to have a little bit more time to see how things developed – a perfectly sensible question. The midwife said the change in heartbeat was only very slight, and she was happy to monitor the situation very carefully, and if the heartbeat was still slow in half an hour, they really should transfer. In half an hour she checked again, and the heartbeat was back to normal. The midwife had the conversation with the husband first but of course in the event of a transfer, it would have been the mother's decision.

If somebody had told the mother in labour that her baby's heartbeat was slowing, what would have happened? She would have gone into the fear response, possibly the whole labour would have slowed down, and almost certainly it would have been more uncomfortable and possibly longer, and generally have been harder for her and for the baby. But because the conversation took place in the kitchen, the mother never knew about it until after her baby was born. An example of a brilliant midwife and a brilliant birth companion.

Lastly, the note finishes: '*Thank you so much for your help.*' This is only courteous, because we can be extremely grateful to the midwife who is with us.

Positions and relaxation in the up stage

You can be in whatever position you like to be in the first or up stage of labour. Many people find being upright and leaning slightly forwards the most comfortable. That might be sitting on a birth ball, leaning on a bed, kneeling in a birthing pool, or standing with your arms round your partner's neck.

Something that is very lovely is the stroking of your arm, as in the stroking relaxation (see Chapter 6), where your husband or partner strokes your hand and arm. Because you have practised it in pregnancy with a deep relaxation exercise, stroking brings a much greater depth of relaxation than it would on its own. And because your husband spoke to you quietly and softly while you were relaxing, then his voice itself is what in hypnotherapy terms is called an 'anchor' for relaxation, and will help when you are having your baby. All these things are helpful.

Gentle back stroking

Another form of stroking that is relaxing and soothing is stroking on the back. The mother kneels on the sofa with her head resting on the back of the sofa, and her husband or partner stands behind her. Fathers, the stroking is done very, very gently with the back of the hands – so gently it is almost as if the fingers are floating on the surface of the skin. As lightly as you can, start on the coccyx, at the bottom of the spine, and slowly and gently move your hands straight up the back, all the way up the spine, and when you get to the top of the back, stroke outwards across the shoulders and then come down the sides of the back. Repeat the sequence as often as she wants. You may find she wants it for a very, very long time because this feels lovely in labour.

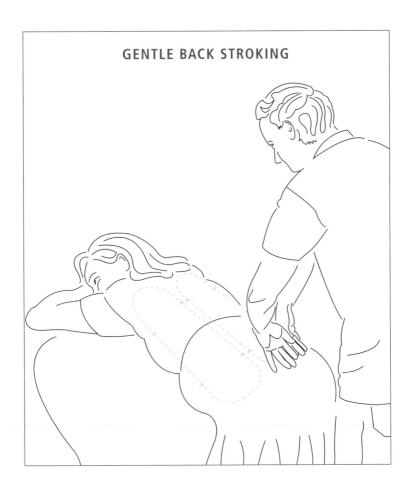

GENTLE BACK STROKING

When you get to the top of her back you can go down the arms to the elbows as well. If you can't reach her back, you can do the stroking on the thighs or the abdomen instead – anywhere. But it is particularly lovely on the back for several reasons. Obviously, you are doing nothing like a normal massage which is pummelling muscles, but what you are doing is very, very gently soothing the nerve endings under the skin, up the centre and down the sides of the back.

When you go up the back, you are soothing the whole of the central nervous system. You are also working in conjunction with the meridian system that acupuncture uses, helping to balance the meridians and the energy of the body. This gentle stroking on the upper back and shoulders also helps to release endorphins – nature's pain relief.

Back stroking is lovely and so simple; a couple of passes up the back has such a profound effect. It is a calming thing to do for each other when you come home from work each day. All the stresses of the day just fall away. In fact, it would be very nice if every class of schoolchildren did it first thing in the morning – then schools would be much happier places.

Natural remedies for use in labour

Some people like to use essential oils in labour, and the one that is known for helping you to relax is lavender, though you can use chamomile if you don't like the smell of lavender. Put a few drops in some water in an essential oil burner and the aroma disperses into the atmosphere, helping you to feel calm and relaxed. If you are in hospital you would need to get an electrical essential oil burner, though some hospitals provide them so you wouldn't have to take your own. Alternatively, you can buy it in a spray to spray around the room.

Flower remedies are also calming. Many people know of Rescue Remedy. My favourite, which is the equivalent, is the Five Flower Remedy – you can buy it online from Healing Herbs. Many fathers put just a few drops in the jug of water the mother has beside her, and once that's done you don't have to think about it again. You can also spray flower remedies around the room. They are very soothing.

You may find essential oils and flower remedies supportive in labour, but they can be equally helpful at other times. If you have had a stressful antenatal visit, or you have to decide whether to agree to an induction, or if all your friends have just called you in one morning to see if your baby has arrived yet, these remedies can help you to remain calm and composed. If your baby has been awake all night and you wonder if you are doing the right thing as a new mother, the remedies can be calming for you and for your baby.

You can also use arnica in labour. Arnica is probably the best-known homoeopathic remedy and is generally used to heal bruising, but it can be used to support any tissue that has been under stress. However gentle your labour, your body will have been working hard and arnica can aid recovery. You can get it from a homoeopathic pharmacy or any good health food shop. Take one little pill when you go into labour, one when your baby is born, maybe one or two in between depending on the length of labour, and perhaps one a day for a couple of days after the birth, letting it dissolve under your tongue.

Follow your intuition

It is also important in early labour to put yourself in the right frame of mind. I'll tell you about one of 'my' hypnobirthing mothers. Shortly before her baby was due she felt that she just wanted to be with her husband, who was working that day in the garden of a big house in the country. So she went and sat in the garden. There was a stream running through the garden and it was a sunny day in early summer. She could have said to herself that, though she would love to be with him, she really ought to do some work to get the nursery ready, or do some shopping before the baby arrived. But she went with her intuition. She sat beside the stream in this garden, reading, and from time to time a fish would rise to the surface and she would watch the ripples flowing out and out until the water was smooth again. Her favourite flower is a peony, and the peonies in the garden were just coming open into full bloom. As she and her husband went home they picked one. She went into labour that night.

She had effectively the perfect hypnobirthing birth of three hours, with no drugs, and was very comfortable. But she had done everything right. She had rested. She had the 'down' visualisations fresh in her mind of the flower opening and the ripples flowing out on the stream. She had set herself up for a good birth. This is what I mean by a mother's intuition. Do what you feel like at all times. It is very important.

A hypnobirthing report and the effect of being observed in labour

I would like now to share with you the story of one couple's experience of hypnobirthing. Their report is interesting on the subject of labour slowing down when you are observed.

I just wanted to tell you what a wonderful experience we found hypnobirthing to be. I make jokes about standing on street corners wearing a sandwich board extolling the virtues of hypnobirthing, but it's not far from the truth. We had our baby girl at home in our little flat with a birthing pool, which took up pretty much all of our sitting room.

I spent the days before her birth preparing our home so it felt really beautiful, filled with flowers and calmness. Our telly and sofas were pushed to the side and the sitting room was filled with my favourite things and pictures. I even got round to making a cake for the midwife. [Always a popular move!]

At about seven o'clock on Friday evening (our baby was due on the Monday) I started feeling surges that were more frequent than the practice surges I had felt all week. We went to bed but I knew that our baby was on its way.

At around 2am I woke up because the surges were getting stronger, and my husband went to inflate the birthing pool. We had had a trial run a week earlier, which was really helpful. We started timing the surges at around 3am, and at 5am the midwife came over to check on my progress. At this point I was using our bed for support, leaning over lots of pillows with a hot water bottle against my tummy. The midwife was lovely, supportive about hypnobirthing and impressed by how well we were doing by ourselves. She gave me an examination, the only one I had, and I think she said I was 3cm dilated.

It was interesting for me to see that, even though I was at home in an environment I felt so comfortable in, with my husband by my side and everything going well, as soon as the midwife arrived my surges slowed right down. I was gently telling myself to stay calm and focused in my own bubble of concentration, but the midwife's presence had a notable impact on me. I could really feel the surges becoming less strong and less frequent, rewinding to how they had felt an hour earlier. My husband spoke to the midwife about this and we decided we would much rather continue with my labour alone, so we could concentrate on getting back into the bubble I needed to be in. The midwife was happy with my progress, and happy to leave us alone until we felt we needed more help. This was brilliant and made all the difference for us.

After she left we kissed and cuddled, and quite quickly my surges returned to their previous length and frequency. At about this point I moved to our tiny loo, where I spent several hours. I had been getting frustrated about how often I needed to pee so it just seemed easier to stay where I was rather than rushing to the loo every 20 minutes or so. Not glamorous but very comfortable. [This is the mother's rational explanation for this, but note that her instinct is telling her to go to a small, safe place, which any female will naturally do ready to have her baby.] *I found the upward breathing very helpful at this point and found myself doing some rather* strange tonal singing, which helped to relieve the build-up of energy. I think this was a really efficient part of labour and my husband was amazingly helpful and was very supportive with my visualisations and breathing.

At 9am our new midwife arrived. The new midwife looking after me was wonderful. She popped her head around the loo door, introduced herself and then slipped away again. She was respectful of our wishes and incredibly supportive of our hypnobirthing. To have her there was brilliant.

I got into the birthing pool and things progressed nicely. My husband was brilliant, I really couldn't have done it without him. My surges were very powerful by now, but I can remember saying to him that I was enjoying it. It's sort of extraordinary, but the reality that we were about to meet our baby was starting to hit me and it was very exciting. The midwife was wonderful when I went into transition. I remember a strange feeling of having had enough and just wanting to get out of the pool and have a break. The midwife helped me to keep calm and not feel afraid of the change.

The second phase of labour was fairly full-on but over pretty quickly, about half an hour, and my husband and the midwife were again brilliant in supporting me through it.

At 1.45am our daughter was born. My husband caught her in the pool and we put her on my chest straightaway. The feeling of elation and surprise was unlike anything either of us could ever remember or could possibly describe. Just 'Wow!' Lots of tears of delight. We waited for the cord to stop pulsing before cutting it, and delivered the placenta naturally.

The midwife continued to be wonderful, looking after us and helping my husband clear up the flat, which really didn't take long. It definitely wasn't the messy event I think I had been fearing – I'm a bit of a tidiness freak.

It was magic to be able to climb into bed a few hours after the birth of our beautiful baby and be in our own calm and *beautiful home. I do use the word 'wonderful' to describe the birth of our beautiful baby, and I know there are so few women lucky enough to do that. I believe so strongly in the power of positive thought and the strength of hypnobirthing. We put in a lot of practice and it really paid off.*

Thank you, Katharine, for teaching us. The gift of helping to give us a wonderful birth is something we will treasure.

It brings tears to my eyes, every time I read that birth report. Please don't think that I am advocating you give birth without a midwife. The couple here managed better on their own only in the early stage of labour, and it would be foolish indeed to give birth without a midwife being there.

Notice that the mother says, 'we kissed and cuddled, and quite quickly my surges returned to their previous length and frequency.' Sometimes I think that when a woman is in labour, particularly in hospital in a strange environment, a father almost feels as though he is not allowed to touch her. A kiss and a stroke are wonderful. Nobody can tense their lips while having a kiss and if your lips are relaxed, so is the rest of your body. So it is a wonderful way of helping a mother to relax while she is giving birth to her baby.

Transition

Then you get to the stage which is sometimes called transition. However, you may not notice it at all. Transition is the stage where your hormones are changing and for a short time your body may not be quite sure whether it is drawing up or bearing down, and so there may be a feeling of confusion. Occasionally I hear this stage mentioned by a hypnobirthing mother, but quite frequently I don't. If you are relaxed and calm, the body can just move easily from the up stage into the down stage.

CHAPTER 11

Your Baby's Birth, and the Down Stage of Labour

'Birth is the sudden opening of a window, through which you look out upon a stupendous prospect. For what has happened? A miracle. You have exchanged nothing for the possibility of everything.'

William MacNeile Dixon,
The Human Situation, 1937

Your Baby's Birth, and the Down Stage of Labour

When the cervix is fully dilated, the mother's body is ready to ease the baby out into the world, but many mothers do not feel this instinct straight away, and midwives will often urge them to start pushing. There are a few encouraging signs that it is just beginning to be recognised that it is better to wait until the mother's body is ready. My feeling is that the body is simply taking a rest before easing the baby on its journey through the birth passage.

There is no rush. The process of birth will always start up again in its own time. If a midwife puts pressure on a mother to breath the baby down when she is not ready, it will only exhaust her and be inefficient. Fathers, make sure she is given the space to take her time and follow her body and her baby.

Because the emphasis is downwards in this second stage, I call it the 'down' stage of labour. For the first stage of labour you use the up breathing and visualisations, to remain calm and relaxed as the uterine muscles draw up during a surge. Now, as you begin the down stage of labour, you start to use the down breathing, as described in Chapter 3. It is a quick breath in through the nose, and a longer breath out through the nose, with no particular count to it. It is a much more focused way of breathing, almost as if your breath is following your baby down. Remember as you breathe that you are not forcing downwards, but focusing downwards. Your husband or partner can help you to remember the visualisations that go with this breathing, gently bringing to mind images that are down, soft and open, like the full-blown flower, the ripples flowing out on a pond, or a small waterfall flowing gently downwards.

Your mind and your body are always working together.

Pushing? – or not

The question that many mothers ask is, 'When should I push?' or 'How will I know when to push?' These are unanswerable questions.

I particularly remember a mother, some years ago now, for whom this was a very big issue. But after the birth she told me, 'It was just obvious from one surge to the next. My primal instincts took over and I just pushed.'

The interesting thing about this birth was that I also heard from the midwife who attended her. It was a homebirth and she was a very senior midwife, because it is often a senior midwife who is sent out to homebirths. My phone rang and there was a woman's voice I didn't know on the other end of the line saying something like, 'It was amazing. Just wonderful. I've never seen anything like it. It was amazing.' I thought, 'Who are you and what on earth are you talking about?' I began to genuinely think it was another form of telephone sales pitch.

Finally she said, 'I was with one of your mothers last night. It was just amazing. I've never seen anything like it. I got to the house and it was quite late at night. Usually when I get to the house and it's a first baby, there's a certain amount of worry and fuss going on and I have to calm them down. When I went in it was completely calm, there was soft music playing, candles burning. They were doing whatever they had been taught to do. I have no idea what it was, but they seemed entirely calm and in control, so I just sat quietly at the side and didn't interfere.' Now this was a good midwife. A really, really good midwife does very little and says even less, but knows when she is needed. She told me, 'They were doing really well, and then when it came time for the baby to be born, it just seemed to slip out. It was so easy. I've never seen anything like it.'

Isn't that interesting? The mother's experience was, 'My primal instincts took over and I just pushed,' and the midwife's was, 'It was so easy. I've never seen anything like it,' and that was a very experienced midwife. Plainly, the mother had been doing her focused down breathing, she had worked with her body, and the techniques had worked efficiently and well.

The only answer to the question 'How will I know when to push?' is 'How do you know when you need to go to the loo?' It's the nearest analogy. First you think you might want to, then you know you need to, and then you couldn't stop it if you tried. It's just like that. Nobody needs to tell you how or when. Nobody needs to stand beside you when you're on the loo telling you when to push – and if you try to push when your body isn't ready, nothing happens.

The old-fashioned way used to be that somebody stood beside the mother and more or less shouted at her, not from any ill-will, but simply because the further a woman goes into labour the more she is in her own place, so you have to speak firmly and loudly to get through to her. It is almost as if the rest of the world doesn't exist for her. The person would say, 'Now push while I count ten. PUSH. One, two, three, four …'

If your midwife starts doing that – fathers, stop her. It is actively unhelpful. The down breathing that we have done works very well. It works on its own. To push with forced pushing of your shoulders, holding your breath with your chin on your chest, simply gets you tired and makes your shoulders ache. It doesn't get a baby born. Doing the breathing and worrying that you're not allowed to push if you feel the urge to bear down can also make you tense up, which is not helpful. So do the down breathing, and then just follow your body.

Benefits of a vaginal birth

The down stage of labour puts pressure on the baby which is thoroughly beneficial. It is like a really powerful massage. It stimulates the baby's circulation, flexes muscles and helps to clear the lungs. Knowing this can be quite encouraging for fathers, particularly first-time fathers who may not have held a newborn baby before and might be afraid they could crush it or break its ribs. When you consider the pressure a baby has been under during the birth process and that its ribs are perfectly fine, just picking up the baby normally would also be perfectly fine.

Also, while in the womb, the baby's nutrition has been provided by the mother and the baby's gut hasn't really been used. Shortly after birth, the baby's gut will be colonised with millions of microorganisms, which are essential to the digestive system and the immune system. During a vaginal birth the baby picks up its mother's microorganisms, to which it already has its mother's immunity, and its gut flora begins to be quickly established. So everything has been thought of. It is a perfectly balanced, almost miraculous process, and the more I see of it, the more I am in awe of the miracle of birth.

Baby – words can't describe it!

And then your baby is born!

One father said: 'Words can't describe how I feel, and no-one who has never had a baby will ever understand.' And that is the very best description I have ever heard of how you will feel.

Skin-to-skin contact

We can't begin to imagine the shock of coming into this world; but we do know that the only things a newborn baby recognises are its mother's skin, the rhythm of its mother's breathing and heartbeat, and its mother's and father's voices. So it is very important for your baby to get back to these as quickly as possible.

A newborn baby doesn't need to be wiped, taken by a midwife, weighed, or anything else. The most important thing is ideally for the mother or father to pick the baby up and put it straight on the mother's chest – no hesitations, but straight onto the chest for skin-to-skin contact. Babies that have an hour's skin-to-skin contact straight after birth tend to feed well. They stay warmer too, and a warm baby is more likely to start being interested in feeding, which he or she will demonstrate by licking or nuzzling at the breast and nipple, or by trying to locate the nipple, sometimes by turning or bobbing the head or twisting the body. These normal responses tend to work best when the baby is skin to skin with the mother so that other reflexes (such as putting their fists in their mouth and sucking them) tend to be switched off. Within about 20 minutes of birth, a baby with skin-to-skin contact will tend to naturally find the nipple on their own, just like other mammals, and it is the gentlest and most supportive entrance into this new world. In the UK we are lucky because putting the baby on the mother's chest is universal practice.

If there is a reason why the mother can't hold her baby all the time – perhaps after a Caesarean delivery – then the baby can have skin-to-skin contact with the father instead, and there is still the rhythm of breathing and a heartbeat. It's still a voice that it knows. The mother and father will also be smelling the delightful scent of their new baby, and the baby will be 'programming' them to love and nurture him or her by this clever scent message.

The first hour is the most important hour of your baby's life.

When to cut the cord

When your baby is born it will still be attached by the umbilical cord to the placenta. The cord will continue to pulsate for a few minutes because the baby's blood will still be passing through it to the placenta, where it picks up oxygen and nutrients and returns with them to the baby. That means that, for a few minutes after birth, the baby is still receiving oxygen from its mother, so if it splutters a little as it learns to breathe, it will still be connected to the life support system it has had for the last nine months – so it has a dual support system for a few minutes. About a third of the baby's blood is in the cord and placenta while this process is working, so if you cut the cord instantly at birth, the baby will lose about a third of its blood. I have been told that early cord cutting can be detected in the composition of the baby's blood for three or even six months after birth. How would you feel if you were suddenly deprived of about a third of your blood?

With the medicalisation of birth, it became normal to clamp and cut the cord immediately after birth. We now realise that it is of great benefit to wait until the cord has finished pulsating before clamping and cutting it, which means that all the baby's blood is back in its body. Even if you wait a minute it is an improvement on instant cord clamping, and two minutes is even better, but it is better still to wait until the cord has finished pulsating, which lasts only a few minutes. Indeed, the latest research shows that it is even better for the baby to wait until the placenta has been expelled before the cord is cut, as the stem cell count in the baby increases dramatically if you wait, and some hospitals have already adopted this procedure.

Some couples opt for a 'lotus birth' where the baby is not separated from its placenta at birth; instead they are kept joined until the structures separate spontaneously a few days later.

The placenta

One benefit of immediate breastfeeding is that breastfeeding is nipple stimulation, which encourages the production of oxytocin, and oxytocin is the hormone that makes the uterine muscles work, as well as being the 'hormone of love' (as we saw in Chapter 2). The uterine muscles continues to work after your baby is born in order to expel the placenta. Indeed, gentle surges will go on for several days or even weeks after your baby is born as you breastfeed, and this is nature's way of helping to get your tummy flat again after the birth of your baby. So everything links in miraculously with everything else, and a breastfeeding mother is likely to get her tummy flat quicker!

The placenta is generally expelled within about 30 minutes after birth. As with everything to do with birth and babies, this length of time is simply an indication and can be very different. A placenta can arrive after ten minutes, half an hour, an hour, two hours. Sometimes the expulsive urge as you go to the loo will help it drop out.

There is sometimes a feeling among the medical professions and indeed among parents too that, once you have had a gentle birth and are holding your wonderful baby, the third stage of labour, the delivery of the placenta, is simply a technicality and should be completed as quickly as possible. But the third stage of labour is a very important part of the process and huge changes are taking place for you and your baby. As in everything to do with birth, it is wise to treat it with respect.

In some places it is almost standard practice to give the mother an injection of synthetic oxytocin to help expel the placenta. There are technical pros and cons with this, and I would suggest that you get the AIMS booklet 'Birthing Your Placenta: The Third Stage' so that you have the facts. The AIMS booklets are factual and give you all the information, and are listed at the back of this book. I highly recommend that you read them.

One thing to consider is that after birth, a mother produces the biggest peak of oxytocin in the whole of her life. This hormone helps with the bonding of mother and baby, and the establishment of breastfeeding. If she has just had an injection of synthetic oxytocin, how will that affect the natural peak of oxytocin, which like everything is perfectly balanced in the miracle of birth?

Vitamin K

The other thing that is offered at birth is vitamin K for the baby. Vitamin K is one of the clotting factors in blood, and the vitamin K level in a newborn baby's blood is much lower than in adults so in some countries an injection is given to bring it up to the adult level. It is given to prevent haemorrhage, in particular brain haemorrhage. It is generally accepted that it makes sense to give vitamin K if there has been any trauma to the cranium during birth: in a ventouse delivery, a forceps delivery, or a Caesarean operation (where there is sudden decompression). It also makes sense for premature babies. But if a baby is of normal size and has been born gently and naturally there is much less justification. Once again you find yourself asking the question that, except in very rare and unusual circumstances, can we trust that nature has got it right, or do we know better? There is not a great deal of research into the effects of giving vitamin K, and again I suggest that you read the AIMS booklet 'Vitamin K and the Newborn'. It gives you the facts, and such research as there has been.

There are various options. You can agree that your baby will be given vitamin K as an intramuscular injection, or that it will be given orally, or you can decide not to have it at all.

The disadvantages of an injection are obvious. You have a newborn baby coming gently into the world and you stick a needle in it. The level of vitamin K rises very suddenly and it is a great deal for a newborn baby to deal with. If the baby has the vitamin K orally, it is the same vitamin K that would otherwise have been injected, and it tastes bitter and horrible so babies try to spit it out. Therefore it is given in three doses to ensure patient compliance.

Or you can decide not to give it at all. I heard recently of one hospital that gave women a form in pregnancy to indicate which of the three options they would prefer – another encouraging step towards normality.

Confidence in a gentle birth

We have talked a lot about practical things, so let's do another relaxation. Settle yourself comfortably and listen to your partner reading this to you, or quietly read it to yourself. Do the long, slow, upwards breathing.

DEVELOPING LIFE

It seems so long ago that this experience began and yet it is so immediate, too: the creation of new life in your body, deep within you, until the moment when you hold your baby in your arms. It seems like a true miracle, and indeed it is a miracle – the starting of life from nothing. And you are the person performing this miracle.

Your baby is already its own small person, moving and kicking inside you. Nature is bringing new life as she always does, and you are the person to receive this great gift as your baby slips gently into the world.

You are experiencing this, and the profound and life-enhancing changes it brings, and your baby too will change and develop in so many positive and delightful ways. These changes are the successful and happy result of these few months of pregnancy.

Your positive and happy state of mind develops and grows as you absorb the knowledge that all is natural and right, and so you become more and more confident, relaxed and calm. And the more calm, the more relaxed and the more confident you become, the happier you are, and this beneficial and self-confirming cycle makes things better and better for you, and for your baby.

Enjoying this experience today helps you physically, mentally and emotionally, and in every way you become much stronger and more confident and powerful. That strength and confidence give you more natural energy, and increase your joy and anticipation of your baby's swift and gentle birth.

You are so relaxed, and completely calm and serene, in your body and in your mind. What you visualise will be,

Continued overleaf...

... Continued from page 183

and you maintain this knowledge and confidence regardless of whatever any other person may say or suggest, because you know with certainty that your birthing experience will be natural and gentle. Follow your instincts. Have confidence in your inner wisdom.

Your birthing experience will be as you have decided, as you have determined, as you have affirmed to yourself. It will be calm, serene and empowering as your body goes naturally through the miraculous process of giving birth to your baby. Nothing at all could be more wonderful than experiencing the miracle of birth.

As your body eases your baby gently into the world, and into your arms, the lessons you have learnt help you to move deeper and deeper into complete relaxation. Your body, your mind and your baby are all working together in perfect harmony, so that all proceeds smoothly and naturally. Your mind is calm and serene. Everything is happening so calmly and smoothly.

Gently and confidently you relax as your body softens and opens. Your baby joins you in this natural and wonderful process, and you both instinctively act together at this very special time, your breath easing and slowing, deep and comfortable, your baby slipping gently into the world where you are waiting patiently and happily to hold your newborn infant.

This is a great natural process and nature knows exactly what to do. Nature creates the surges that flow and ebb in your body like the waves of the sea. Surges, ebbs, flows, all carry you along like the tides on the seashore, like the wash of the sea on the sand. You are carried along by these images; you breathe in harmony with them slowly, deeply and gently. As the sea washes and smooths the sand, so your body is calmed by its own natural, powerful drug, endorphins – completely in harmony with nature, your baby and your own relaxed body.

All is well. All is very well.

As the experience deepens so you deepen in it too, and the deeper you go the more relaxed you become, the easier and calmer your breathing is, the more your body follows its natural rhythms, the more your baby joins with you in its smooth passage into the world.

Relax, relax, all is well, all is gentle, and all is so natural. Allow your body and thoughts to flow with the tide and be carried along in confidence and serenity towards the moment of your baby's birth.

See now that moment arrive. See now your baby coming into the world. See now, where before your body held your baby in safety and comfort, now your arms hold your baby in warmth and love, and your baby's eyes open and gaze into yours.

This is the culmination of those special months of joyful anticipation, of preparing. Now you have brought your baby into the world naturally and lovingly. You always knew you could do it – and you have. You always knew it would happen like this.

You are both so happy and proud as you relax with your baby enfolded in your arms.

All is well.

CHAPTER 12

Practising For Your Wonderful Baby

'A mother understands what a child does not say.'

Jewish proverb

Practising For Your Wonderful Baby

Hypnobirthing works. I have seen it time and time again. By letting go of the fear, negative thoughts and preoccupations your may have about childbirth, you allow the perfect system your body already has to work efficiently and comfortably. Practice is paramount.

You are focused on a calm and natural hypnobirthing birth, so it is very much in your best interests to carefully consider aspects of the birth you want in advance.

Birth plans

A birth plan has two functions. Firstly, it helps you to define your own ideas and research the alternatives so you can choose wisely. Secondly, it tells your midwife how you would like her to support you during labour and after your baby is born.

Midwives are busy people, and they will not have time to read three closely typed sheets of paper, so make your birth plan succinct. Cut out the waffle, the 'I really hope that' and 'If it were possible'. If you put the majority of it as bullet points so that she can see at a glance exactly what you do and do not want, it will make her life much easier and mean that you are more likely to get it. Your midwife wants to support you, so make it easy for her to do so. If you decline certain aspects of care considered routine by health care providers (vaginal examinations, for example, or vitamin K for the newborn baby), it will be easier for your midwife to support this choice if she can justify her actions to the rest of the team by reference to your birth plan. It frees her up to really support you.

Here is a list of all the aspects of childbirth we have looked at in this book. It is not a birth plan, but you can use it as a checklist when you are writing your birth plan.

- **Have your baby** at home, in a midwife-led unit (birth centre) or a hospital
- **Use of a birthing pool**
- **Membrane sweep**
- **Induction** (after the 'due date' or after the waters break)
- **Vaginal examinations**
- **Safe and calm place for birth**
- **Dim lights**
- **Relaxing music**
- **Minimum of talking**
- **Quiet voices**
- **Careful use of words**
- **Artificial rupture of membranes**
- **Breathe baby down** (not pushing)
- **No coaching to push**
- **Wait to cut the umbilical cord** after it has stopped pulsating
- **Wait to cut the umbilical cord** after the placenta has been expelled
- **Skin-to-skin contact** immediately after birth

- **Natural breastfeeding** straight after birth
- **Hold your baby undisturbed** for at least one hour after birth
- **Wait for the placenta** to be expelled naturally
- **Vitamin K:** to be given to your baby as an injection, orally, or not at all.

Practice is essential

For a successful hypnobirthing experience, it is vital to practise the breathing, visualisation and relaxation techniques during your pregnancy. The reports I receive from hypnobirthing mothers show that it was the couple's practice that made all the difference:

'We worked together almost daily before the birth on visualisations and listening to the CDs before bed.'

'The whole experience was beautiful because my husband and I made it that way.'

'I put a large amount of effort into the practice I did at home, listening to your CD, reading aloud my affirmations and doing the relaxation exercises every day for two and a half months without fail. As a direct result I had not only the birth that I wanted, I had the perfect birth.'

'I was terrified from the day I realised I was pregnant. I joined your course, did the homework, and relaxed as much as possible. I guess all the work I did paid off. I am sure it would have been a completely different story if I hadn't joined your course.'

Drawing it all together

The following lists, from below to page 193, effectively define all your practice. I am not saying that you have to do your practice like this; it is simply a framework, a suggestion of what might work, which you can adapt to suit your lifestyle.

Practice is important, but it needs to be done in a way that works for you. The practice suggested takes only about 20 minutes a day as you are a busy person, and if I asked you to practise for two hours a day it wouldn't happen. But if you are able to do more, perhaps once you are on maternity leave, that would be even better.

Daily practice

- **Up breathing,** visualising the sun rising in the sky, blowing bubbles, etc., for two or three minutes morning and evening (pages 42–45).
- **Read the empowering birth statements** and the Colour and Calmness script (pages 87–96). Have them read to you, read them yourself, or listen to them on the *Colour and Calmness* CD.
- **Look at the picture** of the baby in the most usual position for birth (page 55).
- **Pelvic floor exercises** – at red traffic lights or as you wait for your computer to boot up (pages 65–67).
- **Perineal massage** – massaging the perineum and vagina with oil to soften the tissue, from about week 34 (pages 67–68).
- **Down breathing** (can also be done on the loo), visualising an open rose, ripples on a pond or a waterfall (pages 49–52).

The daily practice is a list of six things but they take only a few minutes when you look at them in more detail. You have the upward breathing, the one you use during surges and also for practice, with the visualisations of the sun rising, blowing bubbles, or anything with an 'up' emphasis. A few of these breaths, morning, evening or whenever suits you, is all you need. You will find you naturally begin to use this breathing if ever you are stressed.

Next on the daily practice list are the statements for a gentle birth and the Colour and Calmness relaxation. They are both on the *Colour and Calmness* CD and therefore you just play this as you go to sleep each night. If you are reading them, you don't have to do all of it every night. Just do the part that appeals to you that day.

Then there's the birth picture to look at. I hope this has been put up somewhere prominent in your home by now. The body follows where the mind leads, and this picture puts a positive image of your baby's position in your mind. It has an effect, and looking at it takes no time at all. You just need to remember to notice it as you go past.

There are the pelvic floor exercises, which you incorporate into your lifestyle and do while you're waiting at red traffic lights or for your computer to boot up, for example. Find a time to use an 'anchor' so that they happen automatically. Then they don't have to take extra time.

Perineal massage takes only five minutes. And then there's the downward breathing that you can practise on the loo, but also do it sometimes with your partner, so that you can practise the visualisations as well.

I'm sure that all the daily practice doesn't take more than ten minutes at the most.

Daily choice
(Do one of these after your breathing practice)

- **Head and face relaxation script** (page 81)
- **Stroking relaxation script** (pages 83–84)
- **Calming touch relaxation script** (pages 85–86)
- **Gentle back stroking** (pages 164–166).

Also: squatting, sitting cross-legged, sitting upright, preparing your funny or light-hearted DVDs.
Focus your attention on where you want to be.

Choose one of the daily choices to do each day. The list includes the relaxation scripts you have been given and the gentle stroking on the back. The total practice time is certainly not more than 20 minutes, which is more than reasonable when you consider the benefits it brings.

It is a good idea to practise squatting too, just so that it feels normal if you do want to use that position in labour. Also sit cross-legged sometimes, to stretch the tissue of the pelvic floor and the inner thighs, and remember to be more upright to encourage your baby to face the back. Make sure you invest in your funny or light-hearted DVDs; they are excellent tools.

One very important thing is to focus your attention on where you want to be. If anything distracts you from it, set aside the distraction and resume your focus – because what you focus on is what you get.

When your baby is coming

- **Take your time**, conserve your energy, gently keep doing what you were doing, and at some point start timing your surges. Snack to keep your energy up. Remember to drink water.

- **Watch a funny or light-hearted DVD,** or read a relaxation script.
- **Remember to use** your up breathing and visualisations during surges. You may find some prompts helpful, or you may prefer silence.
- **Call the midwife** or go to the birth centre or hospital when the surges are about three or four minutes apart and one minute long.

It can be helpful to have this section to refer to when you go into labour. Take your time, conserve your energy, gently keep doing what you were doing, and at some point start to time your surges.

Eat snacks to keep your energy up and make sure you have water available. Watch one of your funny DVDs. Remember to use your breathing and visualisations during surges. There may come a point where you find some prompts helpful or you may prefer silence.

Call your midwife or go to the midwife-led unit (birth centre) or hospital when the surges are about three or four minutes apart and one minute long.

Throughout the birth

Mother: Up breathing with up visualisations, moving to down breathing with down and open visualisations.

Father: Protect the mother's space and be her advocate, with gentle prompts, back stroking, arm stroking, and shoulder stroking. Play the *Colour and Calmness* CD. Provide water (perhaps with Five Flower Remedy) and snacks for mother (and for yourself). Prepare an essential oil burner with lavender oil. Give arnica pills (see page 167). The most important thing is just to be there for her.

Enjoy your pregnancy. Remain calm and confident. Allow your birthing body to birth your baby. Birthing and caring for your baby is a natural process of being. **Whatever you do is right.**

For the mother, throughout the birth all there is to do is the up breathing with the up visualisations, moving to the down breathing and the down and open visualisations. It's that simple.

Mothers sometimes worry because usually, if there's something important in your life such as an exam, you revise for it as much as possible, you add more and more, and you produce it on the day. Hypnobirthing is exactly the opposite. All your practice is to let go. The more you practise the more you let go and release, and let go and release. So that by the time you give birth to your baby, you have let go of all the stresses, and the perfect system which is a woman's body can work well.

It can feel a little uncomfortable, as if you are out of control. With most things we do we can take a mock exam, or check how we're doing. With hypnobirthing it is completely the opposite. You do all the practice and you have no way of checking how well it works until you give birth and it does. It is simply a process of letting go.

For the father, his role is to protect your space, physically, mentally and emotionally, and be your advocate. It is very helpful if he can come with you to antenatal visits, particularly in the later stages of pregnancy, because nature programmes you mentally and emotionally to go into your own space ready for birth, so you may need someone with you to have a conversation on your behalf that you could perfectly well have had yourself a few weeks previously.

He also has the role of giving you gentle prompts during your surges if you find that helpful; gently stroking your back or arms, or anywhere that is convenient; and playing the *Colour and Calmness* CD for you. He can make sure you always have a glass of water available with a few drops of Five Flower Remedy in it; he could maybe light the essential oil burner with lavender oil to help you relax; give you arnica pills to support the muscle tissue; and make sure light snacks are available.

The final notes say: 'Enjoy your pregnancy.' Pregnancy is such a very special time. Make the most of it. Remain calm and confident. Allow your birthing body to birth your baby; you can trust that it knows what to do. Birthing and caring for your baby are a natural process of being. Your state of being is far more important than the things that you do.

The last phrase is: '*Whatever you do is right.*' Because you have read this book, I know that you are caring parents. Every parent brings up their child in a different way. Every parent, before their baby is born, thinks they are going to bring it up in a particular way, and then after it is born, they realise that the child is already its own person, and your role as a parent is simply to support him or her in every way you can, to make sure he is safe, to give him all the opportunities you can, and then when you see which way he wants to go, to run along behind, trying to keep up as he develops.

It is the most wonderful and important thing that you do in life, and whatever you do is right. There is no such thing as a perfect parent. Every parent will look back and feel guilty about something they should or shouldn't have done, or could or couldn't have done. But the important thing for your child is your love.

Opposite is a last relaxation for you to enjoy.

STORY FOR CHILDBIRTH

So as you quietly listen to my voice, I want to tell you that hypnosis is simply a learning experience, and we've all had so many learning experiences. For example, I once went boating on a river. This was a place and a time that was special to me, and as you listen you may find that you are drifting off to a place and time that was special to you, that had particular meaning for you. It all began when I found myself climbing from the bank into a wooden boat. I always wondered what it would be like to take a boat down the river to an island. Someone once told me that a beautiful flower grew there, and I always wondered what it would be like.

I set off, not knowing what the experience would be like. I was a little apprehensive of not being on the solid land to which I was accustomed, but my closest friend and some other people who were experienced were with me and I felt reassured and comforted by their presence.

I felt the boat rocking back and forth with each breath, rocking back and forth with each breath, as the current drew it into the middle of the river. I noticed that the river wasn't exactly straight, but wound through the vegetation. And I noticed all different kinds of trees. I saw the sunlight stream through the branches.

The sound of the water gurgling and splashing around me was soothing. I trailed my hand in the water and it felt cool and refreshing. It felt so good as I took a deep breath, and I realised I could just take my time. I decided to just enjoy the moment and took another deep breath, and I breathed deeply and comfortably. I realised that I could be

Continued overleaf...

... *Continued from page 197*

entirely confident: my boat was sturdy, and I was surrounded by people who would take care of me. There seemed to be a calmness as I wondered ... I wondered what it would be like to reach the island and see the wonderful flower I was expecting to see.

So I just relaxed and let the river carry me swiftly downstream ... further and further. The air was so wonderful to breathe in, I filled my lungs ... That's right ... With each breath I took I relaxed more and more. It was a sunny day and I felt warm and comfortable. There was no need to move or talk, so I just allowed my eyes to close, so that I could fully enjoy the experience. And isn't it good to know that we can feel just as comfortable and relaxed, even now? I felt so secure and peaceful that, sitting comfortably, I began to let go of all my worries and fears, all the tension, and simply began to increasingly relax ... all the way.

The river became wider and wider as it carried me to my destination, bringing me closer to my destination each time the current surged. So I just relaxed and let go of all the fears and tension. The river surged and slowed again, surging and slowing, surging then slowing, and each time I became more and more relaxed. I was just happy that I was being carried ... further and further ... towards the end of my journey.

Finally the river ended in a small lake, and I was surprised how quickly I had reached the end of the river. In the middle of the lake was a beautiful island, full of wonderful plants and flowers. My boat was carried right to the shore of the island – all I had to do was relax and allow the boat to be guided by the current. I was so excited, because I was finally going to see the wonderful flower that I had seen in my imagination so many times. I was finally going to see the flower blossom.

I got out of the boat and stepped onto the island. I could hear birdsong, and the sound of the water lapping against the shore. I could feel the gentle warmth of the sun on my back. I walked swiftly along a short, wide, grassy path to the centre of the island. There, in the very middle, was my flower. It was more beautiful than I had even imagined. I held the blossom in my hands, now gently opened into full bloom. The petals felt so soft and tender, and I inhaled its sweet fragrance.

I sat down nearby and just enjoyed the feeling of happiness and joy for a while. I found my mind wandering to enjoyable, relaxing times. Times when I found that I was confident and strong. Times when I trusted in my own body, and in my subconscious to instinctively guide me. Times when I felt filled with love and deep relaxation. Situations where I could allow this energy to flow through me – through every cell in my body. Really focused within me, aware of the strength within myself, of power, of confidence, and those things that we were never really taught as we grew up. I discovered that I could give myself all those things at that moment.

I took my time and enjoyed the feeling moving through my body and permeating every cell. That sense, that feeling that was always there – I just hadn't known it was there.

When I was ready and in my own time, I came back, bringing with me all that I had learned.

(Thank you, Moira Campbell, for permission to use this script.)

As a mother, you have probably come to hypnobirthing for a calm, gentle birth for yourself, and this also means a calm and gentle birth for your baby.

Birth is the most formative experience of our lives, and a baby who enters the world drug-free and alert, to be greeted by a mother who is also alert, loving and confident, starts life and forms its first relationship in this world in the best possible way.

This is the blueprint for all the other relationships the baby forms throughout its life. It has an effect on all of its life and even on all the people it meets. In the long-term, the significance of this cannot be overestimated.

Have a beautiful birth and a wonderful baby.

Katharine

(And keep practising!)

'Do good without show or fuss.
Facilitate what is happening rather than what you think
   ought to be happening.
If you must take the lead, lead so that the mother is
   helped, yet still free and in charge.
When the baby is born, the mother will rightly say:
   "We did it ourselves."'

Lao Tzu, *The Book of the Way*, c. 500 BC

Further Reading and CDs

AIMS

AIMS (Association for Improvements in the Maternity Services) produce many excellent, factual booklets which you can obtain from their website, www.aims.org.uk:

'What's Right For Me?'

'Am I Allowed?'

'Ultrasound? Unsound'

'Birthing Your Baby: The Second Stage'

'Birthing Your Placenta: The Third Stage'

'Vitamin K and the Newborn'

'Breech Birth: What Are My Options?'

'Induction – Do I Really Need It?'

'Birth After Caesarean'

CDS

The following CDs can help you to achieve a calm and natural birth, and to enjoy a confident and happy pregnancy. They are all available in CD and MP3 formats from www.thehypnobirthingcentre.co.uk.

Colour and Calmness – relaxation and positive statements for a gentle birth

Further Relaxations For a Natural Birth

Confidence and Power – releasing fear ready for the birth of your baby

Nurture and Nature – support and relaxation for breastfeeding

Relaxation After Birth

Support For New Mothers

Relaxation and Support For Conception

Suggestions If Your Baby Is Breech

Calm Caesarean

Induction Support.

BOOKS

Here is a list of books that you might find helpful:

Primal Health: Understanding the Critical Period Between Conception and the First Birthday, Michel Odent, Clairview Books, 2002 (2nd edition).

Ina May's Guide to Childbirth, Ina May Gaskin, Bantam Doubleday Dell, 2003.

Childbirth Without Fear: The Principles and Practice of Natural Childbirth, Grantly Dick-Read, Pinter & Martin Ltd, 2004 (1st edition published 1942).

The Thinking Woman's Guide to a Better Birth, Henci Goer, Perigree Books, 1999.

Gentle Birth, Gentle Mothering: A Doctor's Guide to Natural Childbirth and Gentle Early Parenting Choices, Sarah J. Buckley, Celestial Arts, 2009.

Magical Child, Joseph Chilton Pearce, Bantam Books, 1980.

The Farmer and the Obstetrician, Michel Odent, Free Association Books, 2002.

The Caesarean, Michel Odent, Free Association Books, 2004.

Birth Reborn: What Childbirth Should Be, Michel Odent, Souvenir Press Ltd, 1994.

Breech Birth: A Guide to Breech Pregnancy and Birth, Benna Waites, Free Association Books, 2003.

WEBSITES

You may find these websites useful:

The Hypnobirthing Centre

www.thehypnobirthingcentre.co.uk
Read how other couples experienced hypnobirthing. Also for hypnobirthing classes and teacher training.

The Hypnobirthing Association
www.thehypnobirthingassociation.com
For a list of professional hypnobirthing teachers.

Association for Improvements in the Maternity Services (AIMS)
www.aims.org.uk
Provides information on pregnancy and birth.

Homebirth Reference Site
www.homebirth.org.uk
Provides research, information and an online forum.

BirthChoiceUK
www.birthchoiceuk.com
Provides maternity statistics from hospitals throughout the UK.

Independent Midwives UK
www.independentmidwives.org.uk
For information about and lists of independent midwives.

Doula UK
www.doula.org.uk
Provides lists of doulas.

La Leche League GB
www.laleche.org.uk
For breastfeeding support.

Katharine Botanicals
www.katharinebotanicals.com
For natural skincare products for mother and baby.

Acknowledgements

Acknowledgements are generally boring, but mine go to a group of people who are very un-boring. The person from whom I have had most support is Archie McIntyre, who has tirelessly spent many hours advising me and transcribing my notes. Where would I have been without his knowledge and gentle and constructive bullying? To say that without him this book would never have been written is a truism that is true.

Everyone else will be mentioned in reverse alphabetical order to show no favouritism and in a small attempt to be mildly unconventional. I didn't know what a book designer does before I met Louise Turpin. Now I do, and it's very impressive. Victoria and Chris Roads have generously given permission to use the photograph of their family, taken five minutes after the birth of their baby Kitty, on the cover of this book. It looks like a posed picture with models, but it is a genuine hypnobirthing birth. Gina Potts of Zen Birth helped with the proofreading. Jane Pelham struggles with humour and efficiency to keep me up to date, and without her help none of my hypnobirthing classes or teacher training would happen. If every midwife were like Liz Nightingale (Purple Walnut Midwife), there would be many more mothers who could report happy birth experiences. For years she has shared her knowledge with me with great generosity. I am in awe of Jennifer McIntyre's knowledge and experience in editing. I had no idea there was so much to producing a book, and her guidance has been invaluable. Fiona McIntyre has used her talent to patiently produce and adapt the diagrams and illustrations, often very late at night. Daisy Hutchison kindly let me use her birth story, which will help all mothers who read it. Procrastination has been ruthlessly eradicated by Michael Hudson, with humour and occasional permission for time off. Thank you, Alex Graham, for your cover design. I can, at any time, pick up the phone and receive wise guidance from Chris Crossland of Simply Great Copy. His facility with words, as well as his breadth of experience and knowledge, have been invaluable. Thanks to Mary Cronk for permission to use her 'Useful Phrases' in Chapter 9, and to Moira Campbell, the author of the script 'Story for Childbirth' in Chapter 12.

Michel Odent, Ina May Gaskin and Sarah Buckley have kindly allowed me to quote from their work in the chapter headings.

I have learnt from every one of the hundreds of mothers and fathers to whom I have taught hypnobirthing; particularly those who have asked difficult questions that have made me think anew and question myself. My fellow hypnobirthing teachers in The Hypnobirthing Association are an inspiration, not only to the couples they teach, but also to me.

Thank you all.

Hypnobirthing Classes with Katharine Graves

www.thehypnobirthingcentre.co.uk

Hypnobirthing is simple, gentle and profound. Now that you have read this book you might want to find out more about hypnobirthing classes.

Based on fundamental principles and sound logic, Katharine Graves has developed an approach and methodology that is unique and which is now increasingly being adopted and recognised internationally.

Hypnobirthing changes and empowers both the mother and father, and has the most profound, positive effect on the baby which will last a lifetime. The father is actively involved and become an important part of the experience. Hypnobirthing deepens your relationship as you work together for a calm and gentle birth for you and for your baby. You can ensure that your baby has the best possible entry into the world.

Katharine Graves teaches classes in London and has been invited to teach worldwide. She is also available for private classes.

- Discover and release the preconceptions that inhibit a natural birth.
- Release fear, tension, and pain – which can lead to medical interventions.
- Learn deep relaxation, visualisation exercises and birth statements to keep you grounded, serene and positive.
- Massage techniques to release endorphins, your body's natural anaesthetic, are explained.

- Your increased knowledge and awareness put you in control.
- You are more likely to experience a natural, calm, drug-free and comfortable birth – labour can be shorter and more comfortable.

If Katharine has no classes in your area, she recommends the teachers who are members of The Hypnobirthing Association: www.thehypnobirthingassociation.com.

Hypnobirthing Teacher Training Courses with Katharine Graves

Katharine Graves also offers courses for those interested in learning to teach hypnobirthing.

More and more midwives are referring couples to hypnobirthing, and the demand for classes is growing. Being able to teach with confidence the simplicity of a natural and calm birth to mothers and fathers is a privilege and is deeply satisfying.

This comprehensive training programme appeals to mothers, doulas, midwives, hypnotherapists, doctors, nutritionists, and anyone who is interested in making a difference. It leads to professional membership of The Hypnobirthing Association.

It is a privilege to be a hypnobirthing teacher, knowing that you are making a positive difference to a mother's experience of birth and to her baby's life.

'We gave birth to our daughter in April 2012 and it was a beautiful, natural and memorable experience thanks to all the preparation my partner and I put in, including attending your fantastic hypnobirthing course.'

'Hypnobirthing changed my life completely! I turned the biggest fear of my life into the most empowering experience of my life!'

'Hypnobirthing was absolutely the best money I've ever spent and definitely without a shadow of a doubt helped me achieve a calm, relaxed and gentle birth. I strongly recommend Katharine to anyone able to attend her course.'

'Just wanted to say thank you again for all your support in the births of both my children – Katharine, you truly are amazing!'

'I went to your hypnobirthing course last year. I gave birth to a wonderful baby and was actually really looking forward to the day. Now I would love to learn to be a hypnobirthing teacher and share my experience with others.'

'Katharine Graves' approach empowers us all to be able to confidently offer hypnobirthing to our mums-to-be and dads in a way that is sympathetic to them, flexible enough to fit individual needs and reassuring to us hypnobirthing teachers that what we provide is thorough, supportive and presents us all as the professionals that we are.'

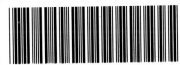
Research skills for nurses and midwives

Note

Health and social care practice and knowledge are constantly changing and developing as new research and treatments, changes in procedures, drugs and equipment become available.

The authors, editor and publishers have, as far as is possible, taken care to confirm that the information complies with the latest standards of practice and legislation.